D0528899

WORK
ASSIGNMENTS
HANDBOOK

THE SOCIAL WORK ASSIGNMENTS HANDBOOK

A PRACTICAL GUIDE FOR STUDENTS

Sarah Foote
Anne Quinney
Matt Taylor

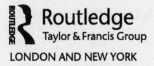

Routledge
Taylor & Francis Group

LONDON AND NEW YORK

First published 2013 by Pearson Education Limited

Published 2013 by Routledge
2 Park Square, Milton Park, Abingdon, Oxon OX14 4RN
711 Third Avenue, New York, NY, 10017, USA

Routledge is an imprint of the Taylor & Francis Group, an informa business

Copyright © 2013, Taylor & Francis.

The right(s) of Sarah Foote, Anne Quinney and Matt Taylor to be identifiedas author of this work has been asserted by them in accordance with the Copyright, Designs and Patents Act 1988.

All rights reserved. No part of this book may be reprinted or reproduced or utilised in any form or by any electronic, mechanical, or other means, now known or hereafter invented, including photocopying and recording, or in any information storage or retrieval system, without permission in writing from the publishers.

Notices
Knowledge and best practice in this field are constantly changing. As new research and experience broaden our understanding, changes in research methods, professional practices, or medical treatment may become necessary.

Practitioners and researchers must always rely on their own experience and knowledge in evaluating and using any information, methods, compounds, or experiments described herein. In using such information or methods they should be mindful of their own safety and the safety of others, including parties for whom they have a professional responsibility.

To the fullest extent of the law, neither the Publisher nor the authors, contributors, or editors, assume any liability for any injury and/or damage to persons or property as a matter of products liability, negligence or otherwise, or from any use or operation of any methods, products, instructions, or ideas contained in the material herein.

British Library Cataloguing in Publication Data
A catalogue record for this book is available from the British Library

Library of Congress Cataloguing in Publication Data
     Foote, Sarah.
     The social work assignments handbook : a practical guide for students / Sarah Foote, Anne Quinney and Matt Taylor.
          pages cm
     Includes bibliographical references and index.
     ISBN 978-1-4082-5253-6
     1. Social work education–Great Britain. 2. Social workers–Great Britain. 3. Social case work–Great Britain. I. Quinney, Anne. II. Title.
     HV11.8.G7F66 2013
     361.3076--dc23   2013006470

ISBN 13: 978-1-408-25253-6 (pbk)

Print edition typeset in 9/12pt Giovanni Book by 71

BRIEF CONTENTS

CONTENTS

ACKNOWLEDGEMENTS

We would like to thank our fellow students who have studied alongside and supported us, and the lecturing staff who share our passion for inspiring and supporting students to become the best social work practitioners they can.

Publisher's Acknowledgements

We are grateful to the following for permission to reproduce copyright material:

Figures

Figure 3.1 from *Experiential Learning: Experience as the source of learning and development*, FT Prentice Hall (Kolb, D.A. 1984), Kolb, David A., Experiential Learning: Experience as a source of learning and development, 1st Ed., (c) 1984. Reprinted and electronically reproduced by permission of Pearson Education Inc., Upper Saddle River, New Jersey.

Text

Appendix 1 Reproduced by kind permission of the College of Social Work (Accessed November 2012, http://www.collegeofsocialwork.org/uploadedFiles/TheCollege/CollegeLibrary/opportunities/professional_practice_development_advisor/domains-within-PCF-May2012.doc) Correct at time of going to press. The PCF is subject to regular updating; Appendix 2 Reproduced by kind permission of the British Association of Social Workers (www.basw.co.uk). Copyright: British Association of Social Workers 2012 (Accessed November 2012, http://cdn.basw.co.uk/upload/basw_112315-7.pdf).

In some instances we have been unable to trace the owners of copyright material, and we would appreciate any information that would enable us to do so.

GUIDED TOUR

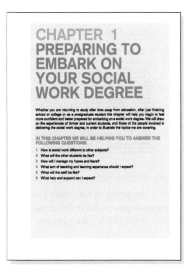

Chapter opening boxes prepare you for the topics to be covered – questions and bullet points explain what the chapter will help you to do.

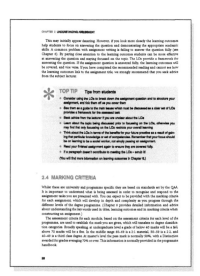

Top Tips from students and lecturers give practical advice on how to tackle different aspects of your social work course.

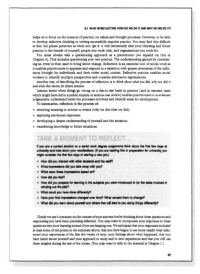

Take a moment boxes ask you to reflect on your own experiences in relation to the topic of the chapter.

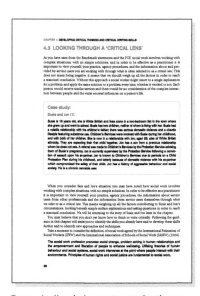

Case studies help you to put the theory into a real world context.

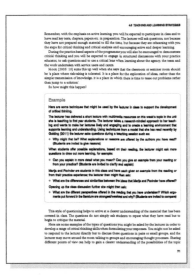

Examples throughout the text illustrate the points being made so that you can see exactly how they might apply to you.

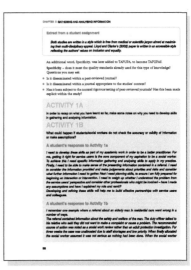

Activities are practical exercises you can do to improve your skills and practise what you've learnt from the chapter.

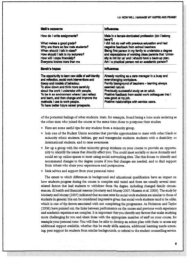

Authors' experiences are great sources of advice and reassurance based on their own experiences as students and lecturers.

References

Further reading suggestions are listed at the end of each chapter and are a useful starting point if you want to explore the topics in more depth.

INTRODUCTION

When Matt and Sara were undertaking their social work degree they realised that the book they would have found invaluable did not exist, so decided the solution was to write the book themselves. After graduation they approached a publisher with their idea and invited Anne, one of their lecturers, to work with them. After many hours working on their computers and many meetings around Anne's kitchen table this book is the result. We hope you will find it an invaluable companion whilst you study for your social work degree, whether you are undertaking this at undergraduate or master's level.

The information in this book is designed to help you to maximise your educational experience. We share the knowledge we have gained from experience and from research studies and offer ways in which you can develop your academic skills in order to become a critically reflective practitioner. However, this information will inevitably reflect our own experiences, preferences and perspectives.

The chapters include extracts from real assignments, and comments from real students who share their insights with you, along with top tips and practical checklists to help you study more effectively. The assignment extracts include references to the texts that were used, but these are not in the references section of this book as it is important that you discover your own up-to-date sources. We refer to the Professional Capability Framework (The College of Social Work 2012) and to the Benchmarks for Social Work (QAA 2008) throughout the book to anchor the material in the documents that are used to design social work degree programme and against which you will be assessed.

We hope this book will travel with you, and support you on your journey to becoming a social worker.

CHAPTER 1
PREPARING TO EMBARK ON YOUR SOCIAL WORK DEGREE

Whether you are returning to study after time away from education, after just finishing school or college or as a postgraduate student this chapter will help you begin to feel more confident and better prepared for embarking on a social work degree. We will draw on the experiences of former and current students, and those of the people involved in delivering the social work degree, in order to illustrate the topics we are covering.

IN THIS CHAPTER WE WILL BE HELPING YOU TO ANSWER THE FOLLOWING QUESTIONS:

1   How is social work different to other subjects?
2   What will the other students be like?
3   How will I manage my hopes and fears?
4   What sort of teaching and learning experience should I expect?
5   What will the staff be like?
6   What help and support can I expect?

1.1 HOW IS SOCIAL WORK TRAINING DIFFERENT TO OTHER COURSES?

The social work degree, whether at undergraduate level or postgraduate level, is an integrated professional and academic qualification and all aspects of the degree must achieve the pass standard. It is a programme of study that is both academically and personally demanding. You will not only learn about subjects such as social policy, sociology, psychology and law, and about social work organisations, but you will also learn more about yourself.

There are some important distinguishing features about the social work degree.

1.1.1 Social work is underpinned by a clear set of values

Many of you will have applied to study social work because you like working with people and have a desire for some form of social justice. A survey in 2002 found that 'the opportunity to make a difference' was the single biggest reason given for choosing public sector work (Audit Commission 2002). You will need to become familiar with the values underpinning the social work degree and demonstrate them in your practical and written work.

These values are set out in the Professional Competency Framework (PCF) and you can find a copy of this in Appendix 1. *Values and Ethics* are one of the nine domains in the PCF, which is divided into levels representing professional development from entry to the degree programme to Principal Social Worker. At entry level

> [s]ocial workers have an obligation to conduct themselves ethically and to engage in ethical decision-making, including through partnership with people who use their services. Social workers are knowledgeable about the value base of their profession, its ethical standards and relevant law.
>
> At this level a social work student
>
> Recognises the impact their own values and attitudes can have on relationships with others
>
> Understands the importance of seeking the perspectives and views of service users and carers
>
> Recognises that social workers will need to deal with conflict and use the authority invested in their role.

(College of Social Work 2012a)

The code of ethics of the British Association of Social Workers (BASW) was updated in 2012 (see Appendix 2) and provides a detailed statement about principles of human rights, social justice and professional integrity and how these must be demonstrated in social work practice.

1.1.2 The experiences of people who use services are of central importance

The experiences of people who use services are of central importance both in understanding the nature of social work practice and in the process of learning on the social work degree. They are usually referred to as service users and carers, but also as 'experts by experience' and 'people who use services'. You will experience their active involvement in all areas of the degree, including selection and interviews, teaching and assessment, as well as in your practice learning placements. There is a growing body of research into service user and carer perspectives that you will come across on your course. Warren (2007) provides a useful introduction to this area.

1.1.3 Social work training develops an understanding of complex human behaviour in social situations

Unlike many subjects, social work theory and its practical application appears to have no definitive answers to questions; ideas are often described as 'contested'. During the degree course you will become familiar with the inspirational international definition of social work.

> The social work profession promotes social change, problem solving in human relationships and the empowerment and liberation of people to enhance well-being. Utilising theories of human behaviour and social systems, social work intervenes at the points where people interact with their environments. Principles of human rights and social justice are fundamental to social work. (IASSW/IFSW 2004)

The theme of *Rights, Justice and Economic Wellbeing* is one of the domains of the PCF. Students are expected to demonstrate their ability to practise anti-oppressively. Social work education and training equips you with the academic and personal qualities to solve complex human problems, where the solution to the problem may differ every time. Social work is not an easy subject to study. Nevertheless, it is stimulating and prepares you for a profession that is varied and certainly never dull!

1.1.4 Reflective practice combined with traditional academic study

Students are expected to demonstrate an ability to write traditional forms of academic assignments which shows their level of independent critical thought and is set out in the PCF domain of *Critical Reflection and Analysis*. Students are also expected to demonstrate an ability to reflect on their practice placements, on aspects of their identity and thought processes, often referred to as *use of self*. You will be expected to include reflection as part of some assignments, presentations and reflective logs.

1.1.5 Practice placements

Learning in practice settings forms a distinct and central component of social work education and training (Bellinger 2010). Students are required to complete practice learning placements of 70 days and 100 days. In addition 30 days of the programme are set aside for practice skills development. Students report that the practice learning aspect of the social work degree is the most memorable part of their experience and is a time when they learn most (Doel and Shardlow 1995, 1996), particularly about values in action and professional identity (Wayne et al. 2010). In other countries the practice placement is referred to as field education or practicum, and you may come across these terms in your wider reading.

1.1.6 The legal context of social work

Social workers have distinct legal responsibilities, and practise within a framework of laws, policies and procedures (see Wilson et al. 2011).

In the *Knowledge* domain of the PCF, at the point of readiness for direct practice you must 'demonstrate an initial understanding of the legal and policy frameworks and guidance that inform and mandate social work practice' and on completion of the final placement you must 'demonstrate a critical understanding of the legal and policy frameworks and guidance that inform and mandate social work practice, recognising the scope for professional judgement'.

1.2 WHAT WILL THE OTHER STUDENTS BE LIKE?

A significant area of uncertainty and concern for students starting the degree in social work is likely to be about the other students.

We can assure you that almost everyone will be asking themselves similar questions. We can also offer assurance that these concerns will be reduced within a few weeks as you get to know your class-mates. Undoubtedly there will be people in the class who are older, younger, more experienced or less experienced than you, and with a range of previous qualifications. This makes for a stimulating and often challenging environment as social work attracts people from a wide range of backgrounds.

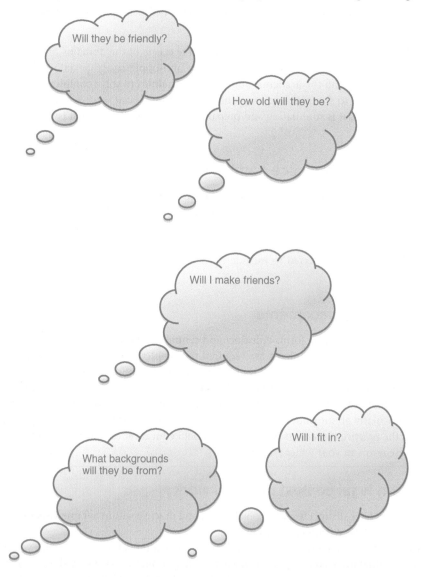

According to the General Social Care Council (GSCC 2010: 5), the previous professional regula-tory body for social work, students on the social work degree have a different profile to students studying for other degrees. For example, in the academic year 2007–8

- over 61% of students were over the age of 25;
- 19% were from non-white ethnic groups (the national population average is 7.9%);
- almost 14% were male;
- just over a third of students reported having caring responsibility for school age children;
- almost half of first year students reported having unpaid caring responsibilities, either for their families or for others.

The age characteristics of social work students are different from those who apply to study nursing or teaching, who are similar in age to the majority of higher education students; the number of black students is higher in social work than in most other subjects; but the number of students with a declared disability is lower in social work than in higher education as a whole (Moriarty and Murray 2007). Depending on which university you are attending (there were 266 social work programmes, some undergraduate and some postgraduate, at 72 institutions delivering higher education in 2008–9), and in which part of the country, your experience may not follow this pattern but you are likely to be studying with students from diverse backgrounds and with a wide range of work, life and educational experiences.

Students from varied backgrounds

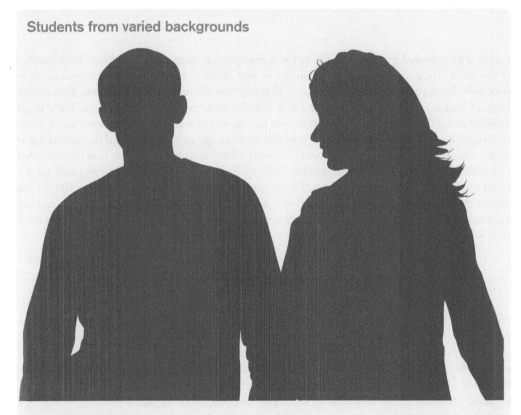

- I'm 31 years old and returning to study after many years working as a care assistant in lots of different settings. I did an Access course at a Further Education College. We studied sociology and psychology and introduction to social work. (F)
- I'm 45, originally from Scotland with school age children and my husband is in the army serving overseas. I did an OU degree and have been working as a volunteer for over a year. (F)

- I'm 20 years old, and have A levels in psychology and sociology and economics. I've been a carer to my mother who's had a mental health diagnosis for as long as I can remember and I've had contact with social workers and the psychiatric services as a result. (F)

- I'm 25 and came to the UK as an asylum seeker. I've been working for a local organisation that provides support to asylum seekers. I hope I can inspire other students to tackle racism and disadvantage and help them be more aware of people from other parts of the world. (M)

- I did a degree in Sociology straight from school and decided afterwards that I wanted to become a social worker after I'd worked in development projects as part of the year I spent travelling and working in South America. I decided to get some experience in the UK and applied to do a Masters in Social Work. I'm 23 years old. (F)

- I'm 23 years old from a working class background with many years' experience of care work. I did badly at school and then did a GNVQ Advanced at FE College. My friends and family don't think I'm clever enough to do a degree but I'm determined to prove them wrong. (M)

- I'm 35 years old and seconded by my employers from my post as a care manager in a statutory social services team. I completed a university Diploma in Care Management some years ago and joined the degree course in the second year. (F)

You may be surprised to learn that the last two examples are Matt and Sarah, two of the authors of this book. These students may have similar or very different experiences and circumstances to your own. What you can be sure to expect is that you will be studying with students from a wide range of backgrounds. This can provide a rich learning environment, helping you to learn about diversity and difference. You may find that your beliefs, or assumptions about people and life, are challenged by other students or by the topics you are studying and you may find this unsettling as it may have an unexpected impact on your personal professional views. Students may feel unsettled and confused when they begin to question views they previously held. The teaching staff on the social work degree work hard to provide a learning environment in which students feel safe to discuss these feelings. However, if you find that this process becomes upsetting, perhaps conjuring up strong feelings about previous life experiences, we would encourage you to seek support from your tutor.

1.3 HOW WILL I MANAGE MY HOPES AND FEARS?

You may be feeling a mixture of excitement and trepidation as you commence the social work degree. Life experiences are likely to have an influence on how you approach your studies, including previous experiences of studying and learning. Factors including gender, age and social class will also influence how you view the academic challenges of the social work degree. Becoming aware of your own thoughts, fears, hopes and dreams and what influences them helps to create a mindset which is conducive to maximising your learning experience.

The mind is its own place, and in its self can make a Heaven of Hell or a Hell of Heaven.

(Milton, Paradise Lost, Book 1, 11. 254–5)

TAKE A MOMENT TO REFLECT …

Write three words that describe you…

Write three emotions associated with undertaking the social work degree…

'Who am I?'
'How do I feel about starting the social work degree?'

You may have written that you are male, female, a student, a parent, a carer. You may have noted a faith or ethnic origin or the paid or voluntary roles you undertake. You may have described feelings including excited, nervous, or curious. The importance of 'knowing yourself' is going to be a key aspect of your social work course as you learn how individuals, including students, lecturers and service users, are affected by their interactions with others.

Whilst starting a university course can be seen as exciting and brings with it new experiences and the possibility of new friends, you may also be worried about being able to meet the demands of the programme.

Matt's experience of starting the degree was that he found anxiety and doubts about his abilities created barriers to learning. He thought other students were more experienced and he worried that he wouldn't 'know' enough.

> Friends and family assumed, and kept saying, that I was going to fail and that I should have a 'Plan B' ready. This led to anxieties which impaired my learning and affected my grades, consequently increasing my risk of failure as I assumed I would fail before I had even started. I was filling my head with thoughts of what I *could not* do rather than looking at what I *could* do. In this way I had as Milton suggested made a 'Hell of Heaven' and needed to change my own thinking as my anxiety and negative thought processes were blocking my ability to develop new skills.

Matt was able to overcome these thoughts by understanding what led to their development. By understanding this he could then identify a plan to both reduce his anxiety and increase his confidence in his academic skills. Matt has developed a checklist to help you reduce any anxieties. This can be used at the beginning of the course to reflect on your fears and to understand what influences them.

HOPES AND FEARS

- Identify the things that are making you anxious about your studies.
- Identify the experiences, past and present, which may be linked to these.
- Identify your hopes for the course.
- Identify the positive influences and networks that you can draw on to help sustain you through the degree.

Anne's experience as a university lecturer meeting new students as they start the degree course is that underneath the excitement and the apparent confidence often students will have specific fears and anxieties. These include such thoughts as: *will I be able to manage the workload ... am I clever enough?* Younger students may be feeling inexperienced compared to the older students who have worked for many years in social care, and students with children may be concerned about balancing family commitments and being a day student rather than living in student accommodation and missing out on the social aspects of university life. To help offset this it is helpful to think about and begin to recognise what your 'script' is. Doing this is the beginning of reflection skills that are essential to understanding yourself and your perspective as much as understanding the topics you will be learning about. (We will be looking at reflective skills in more detail in later chapters, and in particular in Chapter 3.)

Sarah was surprised to learn that Matt saw her as intimidating because she appeared confident in her interactions with staff and had lots of previous experience as a care manager. Yet Sarah's own story is one of feeling both excited and nervous, wondering if she was good enough to do a degree. Her early experiences of education were interrupted by becoming a mother at the age of 15, and her outward confidence masked hidden anxieties about succeeding at university.

These are familiar themes in the work of Collins et al. (2010), who explored the impact of stress, support and well-being of social work students. Be reassured that it is not unusual to feel deskilled and to experience self-doubt.

TAKE A MOMENT TO REFLECT...

- As a potential or new social work student, what feelings do these stories evoke in you?
- Can you draw parallels in your own story in the 'mask' you present to the world and your deeper feelings and anxieties?
- Do their stories help you to consider your fellow students differently?
- Who are you, and what beliefs, prejudices and assumptions do you hold that influence your view of others and your educational experience?
- What skills, interests and prior experiences do you bring to your learning?
- What are your personal values and how do these compare with the values that underpin the social work degree?

Matt and Sarah have both shared some of their hopes and fears about starting the social work degree. They believe that it is crucial to acknowledge your feelings and consider your own barriers to learning in order to make a plan to tackle them. Some of the fears and concerns can be addressed by developing the study skills we present in this book, attending study skills sessions provided by your university or course, and by talking to other students in other years of the course who have overcome their fears. Having come from different starting points both Matt and Sarah developed confidence in their abilities and achieved success. Anne has worked with many students, from a range of backgrounds and with a range of experience who have graduated from the social work programme and become successful social work practitioners.

You may not be feeling anxious about the social work degree and may have enjoyed positive learning experiences before university but we hope this information will help you to be more aware

Matt's concerns	Influences
How do I write assignments? What makes a good grade? Why are there so few male students? When should I talk in class? How should I talk to my lecturers? How will I cope financially? Everyone knows more than me	Male in a female-dominated profession (do I belong here?) I did not do well with previous education and had negative feedback from school teachers Being first person in my family to undertake a degree and expectations of working class parents that 'university is not for us' and I should have a back-up plan. Am I a practical person not an academic person?

Sarah's hopes	Influences
The opportunity to learn new skills of self-identity and reflection, social work interventions and theory and models of behaviour. To slow down and think more carefully about the work I undertake with people. To be in an environment where I can reflect and learn, and then change and improve the methods I use to work people. To have better future career prospects.	Already working as a care manager in a busy and ever-changing workplace. Family background of teachers – learning always seemed natural. Previously successful study as an adult. Positive feedback from social work colleagues that I was good at my job. Positive relationships with service users.

of the potential feelings of other students. Matt, for example, found being a lone male isolating as the other men who joined the course at the same time chose to postpone their studies.

- Here are some useful tips for any student from a minority group.

- Join one of the Student Union societies that provide opportunities to meet with other black or minority ethnic students; lesbian, gay and transgender students; students with a disability; or international students, and to raise awareness.

- Set up a group with the other minority group students on your course to provide an opportunity to identify the issues that directly affect you. You could meet socially or more formally and could set up online spaces to meet using social networking sites. Use this forum to identify and recommend changes to the degree course if you feel changes are needed, and to find support from others who share your experiences and perspectives.

- Seek advice and support from your personal tutor.

The extent to which differences in background and educational qualification have an impact on how students progress during the course is complex and varied and there are usually several inter-related factors that lead students to withdraw from the degree, including changed family circumstances, ill health and financial reasons (Moriarty and Murray 2007, Hussein et al. 2009). The study by Moriarty and Murray (2007) indicated that success rates for social work students are similar to those of students in general; this can be considered impressive given that social work students tend to be older, which is one of the factors associated with not completing the programme. As Holstrom and Taylor (2008) have pointed out, the links between performance on the course and previous work experience and academic experience are complex. It is important that you identify any factors that make studying more challenging for you and share these with the appropriate member of staff on your course, for example your personal tutor. You will then be able to develop an action plan with them to access any additional support available, whether this be study skills sessions, additional learning needs screening, peer support for students from similar backgrounds, or referral to the student counselling service.

Putting this in context

The General Social Care Council (2010) reported that of all social workers on the Register:

- 77% are female and 23% are male;
- 91% of those completing their training in 2007–8 have registered as qualified social workers with the GSCC;
- 70% of social workers are white;
- 16% are non-white; and
- 14% did not declare their ethnic origin.

Whatever background you are from, social work education offers the opportunity to challenge, question and to make a difference. You will meet people from a range of backgrounds whilst studying for your social work degree, and this will contribute to preparing you for employment as a social worker.

From the statistics above we can see that male students are underrepresented within both social work training and the profession. There are a range of reasons for this underrepresentation, including role and gender stereotypes (seeing social work as a female occupation), family financial responsibilities making it more difficult for mature men to return to study, and the public image of social work as not a high status occupation (Christie 2001, Perry and Cree 2003).

Matt's story has parallels here:

My friends questioned why I wanted to go into a 'women's job'. When I started university I was very concerned about not only being able to complete the work because I had found school and college difficult but also how would I get on with a room full of women a lot older than me – and what seemed to be middle class women. I was young and from a completely different world to others in the class. There were only 3 other men. How was I going to make any friends?

Despite his very real concerns about fitting in and being able to complete a degree Matt did pass, in fact he achieved a first class honours degree, and is now a practitioner with a statutory organisation. He made many friends, including people that he thought he had nothing in common with.

Matt had concerns about being from a working class background and fitting in with what he expected to be middle class students. In reality, the socio-economic backgrounds of social work students are more diverse than students in general in higher education (GSCC 2010, Moriarty and Murray 2007). This is a change to the findings of a study by Shaw (1985) which suggested that in the late 1970s social work students were more likely to be from a middle class background.

1.3.1 Understanding other students' stories

As social work students and now as practitioners we have observed that however each person tells their story, each reader or listener interprets the story in relation to his or her own history. The story of your journey into social work defines you and influences the way in which you define others. Story-telling is a powerful tool in social work. For example, you may work with adopted adults who choose to learn their birth story or older people who tell a story of a society without statutory health and social services, of multiple losses and resilience. Each person's story is distinct, as you saw earlier in the chapter.

If you have an interest in narratives we recommend that you read the collected stories edited by Cree (2003) and by Cree and Davis (2007), which provide accounts by social workers, social work academics, service users and students from diverse backgrounds of their motivations to enter the social work profession and their experiences of social work.

Consider the learning a third year student reflected upon when analysing her placement with a statutory adoption and fostering team.

The insight team members have of the impact of their identity prompted a deeper reflection of myself and my impact on interactions. I recognise where my perspectives shape communications, and have developed skills to consider the ideologies of people whose perspectives are either similar or different to my own. I have been able to consciously explore how my past influences my present and this reflection highlights, as Ryan and Walker (2006) suggest, the difficulties some adopted adults may encounter. My learning has included the opportunity to consider the effect of lack of knowledge of one's origins on self-identity and I have gained confidence and expertise in attachment theory, which will fundamentally influence my future social work practice.

TAKE A MOMENT TO REFLECT...

Consider your identity and role, what is *your* story?

● What experiences have shaped you personally or professionally?
● How have other people influenced you – positively or adversely?
● What impact or influence have you had on others?
● What might you learn from this to inform your future practice?

ACTIVITY

Can you 'remove your mask' and share your story with your peers? How could you help others to share something of their story? When Matt and Sarah were new students they found the following group activity very helpful.
Sharing hopes and fears that people bring to the course
Share something of your story that illustrates your hopes and fears, in pairs or threes with your classmates.
You may find this hard, and we are not advocating sharing your innermost fears. Consider reflecting on your previous education, gender or your age in relation to other students. Even this may be hard, but remember that we would expect service users to do the same during assessments, interviews, group sessions or group therapy. By doing this you will begin to develop a trusting and honest approach to sharing. You may also break down the unconscious barriers that people often put up so others don't see them clearly. This will help to remove some of the anxieties and barriers to effective learning.

1.4 WHAT SORT OF TEACHING AND LEARNING EXPERIENCE SHOULD I EXPECT?

Social work education is both demanding and stimulating, and you will experience a range of learning situations. The group and team experience is particularly important, as is the use of personal perspectives and those of service users and carers. Social work students are required to undertake 170 days of assessed practice learning in agency settings and a further 30 days of skills development as an integral part of the programme. When the minimum qualification for becoming a social worker was raised from a Diploma to a Degree, a clear statement about the value of practice learning was contained in one of the underpinning documents: 'Practice is central to the new degree, with academic learning supporting practice, rather than the other way round' (DoH 2002: 1).

A study by Roberts (2011) reported that students, particularly those students who are the first in their family to go to university, often have expectations of the teaching and learning experience that are far from the reality, particularly about contact hours, timetabling, the size of seminar groups, and the delivery of lectures and seminars.

You may have embarked on a university degree with the expectation that you are going to be *taught* and that your role is to listen, make notes and write essays. On the social work degree course, as with other university courses, the emphasis will be on *learning* rather than *teaching* and you will be encouraged to develop active, collaborative and independent learning skills.

Lecturers will seek to impart their knowledge and expertise and encourage students to develop critical and reflective thinking skills. Learning in this way involves students taking responsibility to actively engage with the learning experiences offered. There will be an emphasis on interactive and collaborative learning, supported by the use of technology, with individual assignment tasks and often some group assignment tasks.

When Matt first went to university, he was expecting to be taught in large lecture theatres with tiered seating with a person at the front in a gown talking about their specialist subject. Some of you reading this will laugh, and some may share this image. Some classes may take place in large lecture theatres but others will be held in classrooms, seminar rooms or flexible learning spaces. Lecturers will not wear an academic gown, other than at the graduation ceremony. Sarah already had experience of studying at university so had a clearer idea of what to expect, though she still had anxieties about the people she was going to be studying with and about what the teaching staff would be like.

You might experience some large lecture style teaching but also smaller groups where you are expected to interact with the other students and with the lecturer. Some courses provide an experience of inter-professional education, learning with and about students from other professional groups, for example nurses, midwives, doctors or teachers. In addition you will learn about working with other professionals whilst undertaking practice learning placements. Some programmes use problem-based learning as a teaching and learning strategy, where you will be expected to find out information, often in groups, about a scenario and suggest solutions. You may already be able to consider how these types of learning will foster transferable skills, essential for post-qualifying practice. You will also certainly experience technology-enhanced learning, a term which encompasses learning using computer and information technologies. The course materials are likely to be available electronically in a virtual learning environment, and increasingly there are opportunities for online activities including discussion groups, blogs and wikis and you may also be submitting assignments electronically. This is usually as part of blended learning, where a range of different teaching and learning strategies are combined to provide a flexible learning environment using a combination of face-to-face and online learning activities. It is important to develop your computer skills before you join the course in order to feel confident in accessing online materials and word processing assignments. These are skills transferable to social work practice situations as you will need to be proficient in order to access records and complete documentation.

1.4.1 How much contact time can I expect?

The degree will normally be broken down into modules (also called units or courses). The number of modules will vary but a typical model for a first year undergraduate programme is 6 modules of 20 credits each. The academic year might be divided into two semesters or three terms. The number of contact hours in university-based learning will vary from university to university but might typically consist of 30 hours for each 20 credit module. In addition to the timetabled contact hours you will be expected to read the recommended texts and prepare assignments.

It is important to be motivated and organised in order to make best use of the university facilities to support your learning, including visiting the library, accessing library resources online, attending study skills workshops and arranging and attending tutorials with your personal tutor. In the research undertaken by Roberts (2011) with students who had completed modules in sociology and social policy, a student reported how easy it was to miss lectures and to 'waste' time. It is important to attend lectures and seminars and other forms of teaching and learning, as the material you are currently learning will be of value in other parts of the degree and will enable you to become a more effective practitioner. Some universities may have attendance requirements for all or some aspects of the programme, and non-attendance for students who are sponsored by their employers could be seen as the equivalent of being absent from work without good reason.

Whilst you may not be timetabled to attend university every day during the university-based aspects of the social work degree, during the periods when you are undertaking practice learning placements you can expect to be working full-time. One placement will be 70 days and the final one 100 days. Some programmes may arrange the placement time concurrent with some university-based teaching and learning, on other programmes the placement may be in a 5 days a week block over several months. The programme information provided to you will make this clear, and you should expect an intensive learning experience during the placement elements of the degree, and you will have assignments to produce related to your practice placement to demonstrate integration of theory and practice whilst demonstrating social work values. We will look in more detail later at the types of assignments you are likely to encounter.

1.4.2 Talking in class and asking questions – overcoming your fears

You will have varying levels of confidence when it comes to talking in groups, to other students and to lecturers. It is not unusual to have an intake of 60 students, with seminar groups consisting of 30 students.

Talking in front of a large group can be daunting. Lecturers may tell you that 'there's no such thing as a silly question', but you may still be worried that yours *is* a silly question. The question you want to ask is probably similar to the one many others are thinking about but they don't want to draw attention to themselves or feel 'silly' either. To avoid taking the risk of feeling uncomfortable students often stay quiet. Our advice to you is to ask the questions! Asking questions helps the lecturers share more of their knowledge and experience with you and to clarify any points that were not clear. The lecturers want to help you learn and develop your understanding. You will also learn a great deal from the experience, knowledge and insights of other students. It is important to develop trust and to listen to and learn from the perspectives of other students in your group.

 TOP TIP Some tips for developing a supportive working student group

Develop common ground rules at the beginning of the course (and stick to them).

- Appoint a class representative to attend meetings about the running of the course.
- Meet as a group to discuss issues without lecturers present.
- Always be constructive, professional and polite when challenging the points made by lecturers and other students.

- Participate in class discussions to encourage an exchange of ideas and new learning opportunities.
- Allow everyone to have their say – listening skills are as important as speaking skills.
- Value your own contribution.
- Consider setting up a space on a social networking site for peer support.

Developing skills for working effectively with other students is similar to developing skills for working with colleagues from a wide range of backgrounds and agencies in practice settings. The multi-media learning resources developed for the Social Care Institute for Excellence (Quinney et al. 2009, Thomas et al. 2009, Whittington et al. 2009) on inter-professional and inter-agency working contain information, activities and research findings that will help you develop your understanding and skills. The resources include exercises on assertiveness skills and on negotiating skills, all of which will help prepare you for being an effective member of the group and maximise the learning opportunities available to you.

Baxter Magolda (1992) succinctly highlights the benefits of undertaking education as an adult through a Stages of Knowing model, developed through studies of adult learners.

TAKE A MOMENT TO REFLECT...

Where do you sit within this model?

The model sets out four phases of learning, each associated with phases of knowledge development and a distinct focus. In the first phase the emphasis is on *absolute* knowledge, a concern with seeking 'right' and 'wrong' answers and a focus on 'what do I need to know'. In the second phase the focus is on *transitional* knowledge in which uncertainty can be experiences when there is a range of possible answers, and a focus on concerns with how to make sense of information. The third phase is concerned with *transitional* knowledge, where the learner accepts uncertainty and acknowledges that there is a range of different views. The learner becomes comfortable in this phase with apparently conflicting material. In the final phase in this model, knowledge is recognised as being *contextual* in that it is socially constructed depending on the context and situation. The learner becomes an independent thinker, who can demonstrate critical and reflective thinking.

Students are likely to find themselves in different phases of 'knowing' depending on their progression through the course. You may find it interesting to reflect on this model as you advance through the degree. You may enter the course at the 'absolute phase' and move forwards; sometimes backwards, as your experiences and reflection enable you to grow and develop as a student and practitioner.

Classroom discussions are invaluable for considering new ideas, learning from others and testing out your ideas and beliefs. It is important that everyone joins in with class discussions, as this is a good way of developing the skills you will need when you are a qualified social worker. This can be very daunting in the early stages of university life but if you join in and contribute, even tentatively, your confidence will grow very quickly. Taking part in class discussions is also one of the ways in which you can begin to develop good relationships and friendships with others on your course.

Sarah experienced a sense of belonging by being, as a woman, part of a majority group on the course. This eased some of the anxieties she was feeling and gave her confidence to contribute to any discussion during seminar groups and lectures. Sitting with or near other people you feel comfortable with can provide you with a sense of support and encouragement for taking part in discussion. Try to make the effort to sit with different people to get to know them better and learn about their experience and skills rather than always sitting with the people you talked to or sat with on the first day.

Some assignments may require you to work with a small group of students to deliver a presentation to the whole group, or to produce a shared piece of written work and by developing good working relationships this will be easier to manage. Some students report difficulties when working in groups, but the experience of negotiating with others and handling conflict can develop valuable professional skills in group work situations. It is important to share your concerns with the lecturer if the problem cannot be resolved.

1.5 WHAT WILL THE TEACHING STAFF BE LIKE?

You are likely to come into contact with a range of staff with distinct roles.

The different types of staff you are likely to meet include:

- Lecturers, Senior Lecturers and Professors
- Personal tutors/academic advisors
- Administration team
- Service users and carer educators
- Library staff
- Practice-based staff
- Information technology team.

1.5.1 Lecturers/Senior Lecturers and Professors

A different member of the academic staff team normally teaches each subject at university, according to their specialist area and expertise. One of the exciting things about studying at university is that the teaching staff are also experts in their field, and some may be nationally and internationally renowned. They are likely to be active in research and writing books and publishing papers in academic journals. You may find you are being taught by some of the authors of the key texts you are reading, and some students may have chosen to study at that particular university because of the staff who teach there. The research, consultancy and practice-based work that staff undertake will normally be used to enhance your learning experience by making links between the material you are being taught and the practice realities. Some lectures may be delivered by social work practitioners or teaching staff in a dual role of teaching and practice, and some will be involved in professional activities including advising about policy developments, representing their university or social work education in general on regional and national committees. The teaching staff will each have their own individual style of teaching but all will encourage you to make links between the material they are presenting and the reality of contemporary social work practice. Asking questions will help you to learn more about the topic from people who have a particular interest in this subject.

You may be wondering how to address the lecturing staff. You may be invited to refer to them by their given name, rather than by title and surname, but some may prefer to be referred to by their academic titles such as Dr X or Professor Y. However, despite the informality of using given names it is important to remain professional and polite in all interactions, including email and telephone calls.

You may hear rumours that some lecturers are hard markers and some are not. These rumours need dispelling, as they are normally untrue and very unhelpful for you. Universities have strict marking criteria that must be followed. Markers are required to justify the mark against the marking criteria and to the second marker or 'internal moderator' who reviews a sample of the marking in order to achieve consistency against the academic standards and to External Examiners whose role is to ensure that standards are broadly the same across degree programmes and across universities. However, it is important to follow carefully the guidance offered by individual lecturers about the assignments they have set.

TOP TIP   Tip from students

Lecturers are a valuable resource. An important part of a lecturer's role is to contribute to your learning and development as well as to undertake research and write publications. Use opportunities in class time to ask questions. Always seek their advice if you are not sure about the assignment they have set or the material they have delivered. Book a time to see them individually or in a small group to talk about the assignments they are responsible for and to ask for clarification of the feedback when your work has been marked, in order to develop your assignment skills and subject knowledge.

Individual members of the programme team may have specific responsibilities in relation to teaching and learning, for example as Programme Leader/Director, Admissions Tutor, Year Tutor, Practice Learning Co-ordinator, and you will be given information about the programme structure and staff responsibilities. They may also have research and management responsibilities, for example leading Research Centres, leading research projects or in the role of Head of Department. Do read the programme information provided, which may be a paper Handbook or provided on a data stick or virtual learning environment.

1.5.2 Personal tutor/academic advisor

Normally you will be allocated a personal tutor who will provide you with general academic support and monitor your progress during the degree. They may also be involved in the meetings at the beginning and end of practice learning placements. It is important to be proactive and make appointments to meet with your personal tutor. They are normally the person to talk to if there are any circumstances that are likely to have an impact on your studies, and they will be able to advise you about additional support available.

1.5.3 Programme administration team

These are important people to identify as they are likely to be involved in handling assignment submission and return, registration, and some day-to-day programme administration.

1.5.4 Service users and carer educators

You will experience the involvement in the social work programme of service users and carers from the interview process to assessment, as well as in the delivery and facilitation of learning. Their experience of being users of social work services is central to the programme and prepares students for the realities of practice through listening to accounts of people's experiences and their critique of social work practice.

1.5.5 Library staff

The library staff fulfil an important role in helping you to find your way, physically and virtually, around the university library. A modern university library does not only contain physical books and journals, but also has a vast range of electronic resources. It is likely to have group space for assignment preparation, perhaps with techno-booths where you can work in groups on a large screen. Find out whether the library staff deliver workshops on accessing publications for your subject area, and ask for one-to-one or small group guidance on identifying literature and other resources for your assignments. It is worth investing time in familiarising yourself with the library facilities and with the library website, and finding out how to access passwords to a range of additional online resources.

1.5.6 Practice-based staff

During the practice learning placements your learning and development will be facilitated by a Practice Educator who may be based on-site or off-site. They are experienced practitioners with a particular interest in social work education as well as in social work practice, and have a pivotal role in your learning and professional development by assisting you to make links between the learning during the university-based parts of the course and the day-to-day practice in an agency. They will liaise closely with the university staff and will be involved in assessment decisions about your practice. During the placement you will experience working as part of a team, often drawn from a range of professional backgrounds, and colleagues have a valuable contribution to make to your learning.

It is important to recognise that social work takes place in a wide range of agencies, not only local authority social work teams, but also the independent, private and voluntary sectors. For example, you may be have a placement in a hospital social work team working alongside nursing and medical staff, physiotherapists and occupational therapists, or in a Family Centre working alongside Early Years professionals and educational psychologists. Other possible placements include working in a Women's Refuge, in an alcohol and drug recovery project, or in an arts-based project for children excluded from school.

1.5.7 Information technology team

The use of information technology is an integral part of university programmes, with the use of virtual learning environments for accessing course materials; electronic library resources; and the use of technologies in teaching and learning activities. You will be expected to word process your assignments and to access online materials. The information technologists will normally provide support for university computer and printing facilities and advice about programme-related technology issues.

1.6 WHAT OTHER HELP AND SUPPORT CAN I EXPECT?

1.6.1 The student group can provide an effective support network

You will find that there is a wealth of knowledge within your group, which might include experience of writing assignments or of social work and social care organisations. In addition to being a source of knowledge and experience the group can provide moral support and a safe 'sounding off' space. We recommend that you form study groups and identify study partners (sometimes called study buddies) to help you generate ideas, test out your understanding of topics you are covering, and formulate arguments.

Study partners (or study buddies) were essential for both Matt and Sarah, who believe this helped them to achieve good grades by reinforcing their commitment to be active learners by discussing the content of lectures, class activities and the literature they were reading. Students are increasingly using social networking sites to provide academic support and to arrange social activities, as well as providing a way to share experiences about their studies.

There may be formal *peer support systems* available, often with students from another year acting as peer mentors to students, and there may be peer support schemes to support students from minority groups in order to share experiences and offer practical advice and emotional support. One example we are aware of is a peer support group for Black and Minority Ethnic students on a programme in a predominantly white area of the country (Calvin Thomas and Howe 2011).

You will be asked to elect a *student representative* from the student group, who will attend programme meetings and speak on behalf of the student year-group. Training may be provided by the Students Union and engaging in this role can enhance future job applications by demonstrating experience of the responsibilities of undertaking committee work and advocating on behalf of other students.

TOP TIP   Finding a good 'study buddy'

Remember that a good friend does not always make a good study partner.

- You might want to find someone who thinks in a similar way as you or someone who thinks differently – try both and see what works.
- Don't rule out having a study partner if it hasn't worked for you in the past, you may simply not have found the right person.
- Consider forming a study group and sharing books and other resources.
- Try and find someone whose timetable and working patterns fit yours.
- Use different media such as phone, email or social networking sites to discuss your ideas.
- Keep checking that the arrangement works for both of you – the idea of study partners is to help both people.

1.6.2 Study skills support

The university where you are studying will provide study skills support, and we strongly encourage you to find out about it and use this service. Check in your course handbook, the course website and with teaching staff to see what is available. For students with a specific learning need, for example those with dyslexia, there will be specific support available.

The experience of a student diagnosed with dyslexia:

> I was worried that I was making a huge mistake by attempting to complete a degree and that I would be out of my depth academically. My anxiety and fear stemmed from all my experiences of education, in school and then in my adult life, where my academic work was never quite good enough however hard I tried. I had not had a formal diagnosis of dyslexia until this was offered to me at university. The support and resources provided helped me to develop strategies and my confidence and marks increased.

These are the words of another social work student who achieved a first class honours degree. She was diagnosed as having dyslexia and used the support services available at her university to develop study habits that worked well for her and led to high achievements.

Here is some sound advice from social work students diagnosed as having additional learning needs.

- Access any support services that are available, and do remember that the staff are not there to give you the answers to questions set in assignments but to help *you* give your answers the best way you can.
- Apply for the Disabled Student Allowance if you meet the criteria to ensure you have the additional support and equipment you need to be able to study effectively.
- Ensure you follow any additional procedures for submitting work that have been advised as part of the support for your particular learning need.
- Consult your personal tutor for advice and support in areas of study you find difficult.
- Read the lecture notes and other class resources provided in advance of the class on the virtual learning environment.
- Make sure you have a clear understanding of the expectations of each assignment. Ask for clarification from the lecturers to ensure that you have understood correctly.
- Invest time in becoming familiar with any equipment and computer software that may have been provided.
- Have copies of any assessments in connection to your learning need diagnosis available for practice teachers and placement supervisors to assist them in providing suitable support when you are on placement.
- Celebrate what you achieve and believe in what you have done.
- Be proactive and take responsibility for your learning.
- Know your time management and learning styles and use them to help you study more effectively.
- Make use of social networking sites set up by fellow students to provide informal support.

TOP TIP   Top tips for your assignments

Of course, we recognise that your initial fears and anxieties may focus on passing your assignments and this is likely to be the main reason why you have been drawn to this book. To allay your current fears try to incorporate the following tips from students into your preparation for learning.

TOP TIP   Preparing to succeed – tips from social work students

Read your course handbook and begin to find your way round the university website and virtual learning environment. Make notes on what you don't understand and ask questions about what isn't clear to you.

- Develop confidence in computer skills before you start the course.
- Make an appointment to spend time with your personal tutor. They will become an important part of your support network and can help you understand the course expectations. Take up offers of individual and group tutorials – these will help you to learn more about the course and provide an opportunity to discuss your fears and anxieties and pick up tips for success.

- Attend the library tour and induction, study skills support classes and any social opportunities to begin getting to know the other students and making friends.

- Take your learning opportunities seriously. This might mean turning down social arrangements with friends doing courses which seem to make fewer demands on their time.

- Plan your time very carefully. Using a wall planner or diary helps with keeping on top of deadlines. Keep ahead of yourself where possible. Some students will need to consider how to juggle home and university life, others how to juggle study and employment, and others how to juggle socialising and study. Remember the importance of taking time out to ensure you have a healthy balance.

- Don't book in any social engagements just before an essay is due in – you'll relax better if you've handed in your assignment.

- Buy a notebook and begin to make daily notes on your thoughts and feelings. Later you can try to make sense of these using the reflection tools and techniques that you'll be introduced to.

- Talk to other students about planning essays – you'll all benefit from trying to put your ideas into words, but don't copy!

- Don't turn up late to lectures: you won't be popular with lecturers or other students.

- Dedicate plenty of time to planning, researching and writing assignments; never leave it to the last minute.

- And finally – if you really want high grades, be prepared to work very hard. Both Matt and Sarah approached the degree with the same commitment they would make to a full-time job. For Sarah this meant 9–5, Monday to Friday, either in the library or in lectures/class. For Matt it meant working into the small hours most evenings when he would have preferred to have been in the pub.

Further tips from students and staff can be found in the Teaching and Learning Guides produced by the social policy and social work subject centre (SWAP 2007).

CONCLUSION

We hope you feel better prepared to embark on your social work degree. The other chapters in this book will guide you towards successful assignment writing for social work, by considering what is assessment, how to develop reflection and reflective writing, how to develop critical thinking and writing skills, how to analyse information and how to plan and construct an assignment. We wish you well on your journey through the degree programme.

FURTHER READING

Cree, V. (Ed) 2003. *Becoming a social worker*. Abingdon: Routledge.

Warren, J. 2007. *Service user and carer participation in social work*. Exeter: Learning Matters.

CHAPTER 2
UNDERSTANDING ASSESSMENT

In this chapter we will introduce you to some key study skills concepts and terms associated with assignments to help you develop familiarity and confidence with the language of academic assignment writing. This will include the generic language and the subject-specific language used in setting assessments, and understanding these will help you to demonstrate your understanding of social work knowledge, values and skills, and the issues, discourses and arguments associated with them. We aim to help you navigate through what might initially seem like a maze of unfamiliar words and concepts.

IN THIS CHAPTER WE WILL:

1 Explain the purposes of assessment.

2 Clarify different types of assessment.

3 Introduce learning outcomes.

4 Familiarise you with assessment criteria.

5 Introduce you to academic protocol.

6 Provide advice on understanding and acting on feedback.

2.1 THE PURPOSES OF ASSESSMENT IN SOCIAL WORK EDUCATION

On the social work degree you will be formally assessed on both your university-based and practice-based learning: both are essential elements of the integrated academic and professional qualification. Assessment has been described as 'a critical component of social work education … with a vital role to play' (Green Lister et al. 2005, 693) and as 'one of the principal drivers of student learning; the examinations and essays which [lecturers] set have a major impact on how, and indeed what, students learn' (Cree 2000, 189). Assignments have several purposes. They are designed to test your knowledge and understanding of the subjects you are learning about and provide an opportunity to receive feedback on your progress along with detailed constructive and developmental comments which can be used to improve your assignment writing skills and your understanding of social work. The analytical skills involved will prepare you for making clear judgements in your professional practice.

Assignments are intended to be effective, efficient, inclusive and sustainable (Hudson 2010) and to engage students with the issues and practices of the discipline being studied. Students are expected to demonstrate knowledge, insight and understanding of social work. Academic writing is formal, and in that sense different from everyday writing.

The Benchmarks for Social Work (QAA 2008: para. 6.7) explain that

the purpose of assessment is to:

- provide a means whereby students receive feedback regularly on their achievement and development needs
- provide tasks that promote learning, and develop and test cognitive skills, drawing on a range of sources including the contexts of practice
- promote self-evaluation, and appraisal of their progress and learning strategies
- enable judgements to be made in relation to progress and to ensure fitness for practice, and the award, in line with professional standards.

As you can see from this list, assessment involves much more than testing and grading your knowledge and understanding at any given point, it is an integral part of the learning experience of becoming a social worker. It is important to note that self-evaluation of your own learning is important throughout the social work degree and prepares you for engaging in continuous professional development during your social work career. We acknowledge that assessment can be experienced as stressful and demanding, but it can be less stressful if you understand more about the purpose and process of assessment. Assessment can determine what students consider to be important on their programme, and the types of assessment experienced will influence how students learn (Cree et al. 2006) but, as Singh has pointed out (2001), it is important not to simply focus exclusively on what is being assessed, but on the holistic experience of the social work degree. What might seem like a sound strategic approach can result in partial learning and a competitive rather than collaborative learning experience.

Studies by Worsley et al. (2009) and by McCann and Saunders (undated) describe how previous experiences of assessment may be very different to what will be experienced on the social work degree.

TAKE A MOMENT TO REFLECT …

- What are your previous experiences of assessment?
- What are your expectations of assessment on the social work degree?

Whilst you are studying for a social work degree you are expected to be self-motivated and to develop into an independent learner. In a guide for students with contributions from social work and social policy students a student commented that 'lecturers should also encourage autonomy in students by teaching them how to work for themselves and ensure that they have sufficient knowledge and skills to be successful' (SWAP 2008).

Both Worsley et al. (2009) and McCann and Saunders (undated) reported that students identified the challenge of making an adjustment to becoming a more independent learner as greater if they had previously been used to a more directive and structured learning experience with all the information provided. In addition, some master's students had experienced very different assessment styles, for example if they had undertaken a fine arts or science degree and had to adjust to new forms of assessment as well as a new subject area.

As the social work degree is a combined academic and professional award the assessment strategies developed by the programme team will be relevant to social work practice, to theories for and about social work and will involve a range of assessment tasks.

We hope that the information in this chapter will help you to understand more clearly the role of assessment in the social work degree, to help manage your expectations of assessment and to smooth the transition from school, college or another university programme.

2.2 DIFFERENT TYPES OF ASSESSMENT

Learning on the social work programme involves a focus on both the process of learning and the content of the curriculum.

- Awareness raising, skills and knowledge acquisition
- Conceptual understanding
- Practice skills and experience
- Reflection on performance (QAA 2008).

You will be assessed many times, using a variety of formats and by a range of people including lecturers, service users and carer educators, practice-based staff and possibly by other students. As well as the wide range of learning activities that you read about in Chapter 1, the range of assignments will include essays, reports, individual and group presentations, posters, portfolios of work relating to practice learning, and on master's programmes you are likely to be writing a dissertation. There has been in recent years an increase in the use of technology-enhanced learning and alongside that an increase in technology-enhanced assessment. The assignments overall are designed to enable you to develop and demonstrate the skills that underpin professional judgement.

> What is important to bear in mind is that assignments and assessment should be seen as 'an integrated part of the learning process, clearly linked to learning outcomes, rather than just a series of hurdles to be jumped and forgotten'.
>
> (Rust 2007: 128)

Assignments can be *formative* or *summative*.

2.2.1 Formative assignments

Formative assignments are often set early in the programme to provide an opportunity to attempt or practise academic writing and to gain feedback, without the mark or grade awarded 'counting' towards academic credit. They can also be used throughout the programme to enable students to gain rapid feedback and monitor progress. You may find this referred to as assessment *for* learning, as opposed to assessment *of* learning. Some examples of formative assessment follow.

Example 1

As part of 'learn to learn' activities at the start of an undergraduate social work programme, students are assigned to groups and prepare a poster and a short presentation. Themes included are 'what are social work values?', 'what is anti-oppressive practice?' or 'what is social work assessment?'. This is used as an ice-breaking activity and to develop confidence, facilitate group cohesion and help students engage early with some key concepts about social work. Verbal and written developmental feedback is provided by lecturers, and students have reported that this is a very useful learning experience.

Example 2

As part of a year 1 module, students write a 1000-word essay which is marked against the expected standard for this level of the programme, detailed written and verbal feedback is provided along with an indicative grade. This mark does not count towards academic credit for the unit but students are required to complete the essay. This provides the opportunity to practise academic writing, including learning how to reference sources using the university's specific referencing format. It also provides an opportunity to identify strengths and weaknesses in academic writing and to signpost students to academic writing workshops and online study skills resources. A further assignment is then completed on a different topic, for which the marks 'count'.

Example 3

Students in a second year module complete an individual weekly blog. Feedback is provided by the module team for this formative activity. The blog contents are then amalgamated and edited by the students in order to contribute to a final assessed group blog.

Example 4

During lectures for a unit which develops research awareness multiple-choice questions are presented and students use individual voting pads to choose the correct answer. The responses are immediately calculated and displayed on the screen in the lecture theatre in order for students to see the correct answer and compare it to their answer, and the lecturer is able to gain immediate feedback on which areas of the curriculum the students are most or least competent in. Students take an online multiple-choice exam as part of the summative assessment and the voting pads activities can provide feedback on areas where more revision is needed (see Hutchings et al. 2012, Pulman et al. 2012).

Example 5

A research tool (the questionnaire used to gather information) developed as part of a research project which considered how students develop confidence in research skills was also used as an ongoing formative assessment activity by students who were able to use it to monitor their own progress (Quinney 2008, Quinney and Parker 2010).

Formative assignments are helpful, depending on the format used, in the following ways:

- to develop confidence in assessment tasks;
- to gain feedback on understanding;
- to gain feedback on academic skills development and progress;
- to identify areas of strengths and weaknesses;
- to develop personal study plans.

They are a useful way of adjusting to the type and format of assignments on the programme, becoming familiar with the language of learning outcomes and assessment criteria. Some students approach their studies with an expectation that the subject areas contain certainty and facts, wrong or right answers, but the reality is that social work is not an area where there are certainties, and social work education aims to prepare students for uncertainty and complexity (Taylor and White 2006). This requires the development of critical analysis and critical reflection (we explore these themes in detail in Chapter 3 and Chapter 4).

Formative assessments are also useful to lecturers as they gain insight into student progress and identify areas which need further input, and adjustments can be made to the teaching and learning curriculum as a result (Quinney 2008).

2.2.2 Summative assignments

These are assignments where the mark or grade awarded 'counts' towards academic credit. A selection of assignment formats follows; the list is by no means exhaustive and may include assignments produced in formative assessment tasks.

Presentations

You are likely to experience an assignment that involves working in groups, or individually to gather and present material to the class. This involves a range of skills including knowledge of the topic, the ability to use creative formats to enhance understanding, and effective communication

TOP TIP   Tips from students

If using PowerPoint or a similar computer programme check that the size and colour of the chosen font can be read by the audience, including those sitting at the back. If possible rehearse in the room where you will be presenting – checking that you know how to operate any technology equipment. Back up your presentation on a memory stick, bring a paper copy, set out the room and remember to have water to hand as nerves can lead to a dry mouth. Make a conscious effort to talk slowly as nerves can lead you to speeding up your delivery.

skills that engage and persuade your audience. Presentations can be daunting but become less so with repetition, practice and confidence in your subject knowledge and communication skills. Presenting ideas to an audience is an important range of skills to develop as it will be required in practice settings, particularly in team meetings, funding panels and case conferences.

Essays

Essays provide the opportunity to search for information, collate the information, analyse the material and develop a sound and coherent written argument which addresses the assignment question. As the social work degree has a central focus on social work practice, the essay may require you to use practice examples to illustrate the points you are making and to demonstrate how the learning can be applied to practice situations. Chapter 6 explores in detail the process of information gathering, planning and writing an assignment.

Portfolios

Portfolios are a common form of gathering evidence of your learning and skills during practice learning placements. They are likely to include accounts of direct observations of your practice, critical incident analyses, reflective logs, evaluation of your learning and identification of future learning needs, feedback from service users and carers and other professionals. The programme on which you are studying will provide detailed information about the contents of the portfolio. A detailed guide to developing your practice learning portfolio is provided in the book written by Fenge et al. (2012). As the QAA (2008: para. 6.10) points out, practice is assessed 'not as a series of discrete practical tasks, but as an integration of skills and knowledge with relevant conceptual understanding'.

Reports

As an alternative to a formal essay you may be required to produce a report as an assignment. This is used to introduce extended writing tasks similar to those that may be required in professional practice situations.

Posters

These are an effective way of summarising key points of learning in a format that has visual impact. Presenting the poster to the class or panel of assessors provides the opportunity to practise skills in summarising and disseminating complex ideas in an accessible and compact format. The skills demonstrated are similar to those used when presenting information to a team meeting or at a professional development event such as a conference.

Child observations

This form of assessment may be part of a module that includes learning about development across the lifespan. You may be required to observe a young child for a period of time, noting their behaviour and interactions and writing a critique of this based on your learning about child development.

Exams

Exams are not a common feature of social work programmes and consequently not all undergraduate or postgraduate courses have examinations as a form of assessment. Exams can take many different formats including multiple choice or essay style. They may be handwritten or take place in a computer room. Some allow students to access literature during the exam; some expect students to rely on their memory. In a study by Hutchings et al. (2012) the majority of students reported that they preferred an exam to writing an essay.

Dissertations or extended study

Particularly at master's level you are likely to be producing an extended in-depth piece of work, using systematic and rigorous literature search in the form of a literature review or, if ethics approval processes permit, by gathering original data. A precursor to the dissertation, project or extended essay is a 'proposal', an assignment that sets out the scope, the focus and the methodology. It is important to be familiar with online searching of the library resources using a range of databases. There are several useful texts that support dissertation writing and you will be guided and supported by a dissertation supervisor, and possibly a peer group of other students who are interested in a similar theme or similar approach.

2.3 LEARNING OUTCOMES

These are a series of statements about what a student is expected to know and to demonstrate this in an assessed piece of work. Alongside answering the main question students must explicitly demonstrate that they have met the learning outcomes (LOs) by demonstrating learning. Learning outcomes serve two main purposes: firstly they enable a student to recognise what they need to demonstrate in their assignment and, secondly, they give lecturers a consistent framework against which to assess the content of the assignment.

Concerns about understanding the learning outcomes can, in our experience, cause initial confusion about their meaning as they are often written in 'university-speak' rather than everyday language. It is important to establish that you understand the terminology being used, asking for clarification from the lecturer who is teaching the module to which they apply. Do not be afraid to ask, as rather than 'making a fool of yourself' as you may fear, the other students in the class are very likely to be grateful to you for asking the question that they have not felt confident to ask themselves.

Learning outcomes are normally set out as a list of criteria which must be demonstrated in assignments. They provide students with the opportunities to highlight the learning they have achieved, and can provide a structure for the assignment. The learning outcomes will normally accompany the assignment question, title or task, and should guide your assignment writing.

Example The assignment briefing may take the following form

Title

Critically explore the impact that the Fairer Access to Care (FAC) criteria has had on statutory social work within Adult Social Care services. How do these criteria fit with social work values and anti-oppressive practice?

Learning outcomes

1. Discuss the legal framework within adult social care services.
2. Critically explore some of the circumstances when Fairer Access to Care criteria apply to service users and carers.
3. Highlight some of the main issues faced by social workers when implementing social care policy.
4. Debate the importance of a well-developed social work skills base.

This may initially appear daunting. However, if you look more closely the learning outcomes help students to focus on answering the question and demonstrating the appropriate academic skills. A common problem with assignment writing is failing to answer the question fully (see Chapter 6). By paying close attention to the learning outcomes students can be more effective at answering the question and staying focussed on the topic. The LOs provide a framework for answering the question. If the assignment question is answered fully, the learning outcomes will be covered, and vice versa. If you have completed the recommended reading and cannot see how the learning outcomes link to the assignment title, we strongly recommend that you seek advice from the subject lecturer.

TOP TIP   Tips from students

- Consider using the LOs to break down the assignment question and to structure your assignment, and tick them off as you cover them

- See them as a guide to the main issues which must be discussed as a clear set of LOs provides a framework for the assessed task

- Seek advice from the lecturer if you are unclear about the LOs

- Learn about the topic being discussed prior to focussing on the LOs, otherwise you may find that only focussing on the LOs restricts your overall learning

- Think about the LOs in terms of the benefits for your future practice as a result of gaining that particular knowledge or set of competencies. Remember that your focus should be on learning to be a social worker, not simply passing an assignment.

- Read your finished assignment again to ensure they are covered fully.

- If a paragraph doesn't contribute to meeting the LOs – scrub it!

(You will find more information on learning outcomes in Chapter 6.)

2.4 MARKING CRITERIA

Whilst these are university and programme specific they are based on standards set by the QAA. It is important to understand what is being assessed in order to recognise and respond to the assignment tasks you are presented with. You can expect to be provided with the marking criteria for each assignment, which will develop in depth and complexity as you progress through the different levels of the degree programme. (Chapter 6 provides detailed information and advice about understanding the key words used in titles, learning outcomes and in marking criteria when constructing an assignment.)

The assessment criteria for each module, based on the assessment criteria for each level of the programme, are used to establish the mark you are given, which will translate to degree classification categories. Broadly speaking, at undergraduate level a grade of below 40 marks will be a fail, above 70 marks will be a first. In the middle range 60–69 is a 2:1 material, 50–59 is a 2:2, and 40–49 is a third class degree. At master's level the pass mark is normally 50%, with a Distinction awarded for grades averaging 70% or over. This information is normally provided in the programme handbook.

Generic assessment criteria provide clarity and consistency for markers. At one university the generic assessment criteria consists of four areas: subject knowledge and understanding, intellectual skills, subject-specific skills and transferable skills, which are consistent with the categories set out in the subject benchmarks. A range of expectations about performance in each category are set out for each mark range.

A useful exercise is to consider what mark or grade you think you should be awarded and why. What feedback would you give yourself? This helps to develop an appraisal of your own abilities against the criteria provided and to identify any gaps in your knowledge or academic writing skills.

Assignments will be marked by a named member of the programme team and there will be a system of moderation, or second marking, to ensure that the marking is fair and consistent. The moderation of marks involves External Examiners. External Examiners are independent subject specialists appointed by the programme to oversee internal university marking and validate standards. External markers are usually experienced academics from another university; they monitor assessment standards throughout the course. This involves scrutinising a selection of assignments from each module, including assignment work associated with practice portfolios, and providing feedback to the programme team. They attend the Board of Examiners meeting during which formal decisions are made about grades, progression to the next stage and degree classification.

2.5 ACADEMIC WRITING PROTOCOL

Learning about the principles and practices of academic assessment may form part of a study module at the start of the programme of study. It may include sessions on information retrieval (using the electronic library resources), about referencing, plagiarism, essay writing skills and presentation skills. You may also have the opportunity to see and to read work produced by other students, who have given permission for their work to be used in this way. This can help to dispel concerns about assignment writing and help you to feel reassured that it is possible to gain good marks and that the assignment is less complicated than you had imagined.

2.5.1 Style

There are rules about the style of academic assignment writing. It is essential to write using full sentences and formal language (rather than the informal everyday style of communication which uses colloquial terms and shortened versions of words and phrases). Proper punctuation and grammar must be used, and the work set out using full paragraphs and with a clear structure. (This is explained more fully in Chapter 6.)

2.5.2 Plagiarism

In its most basic form plagiarism is intellectual theft. It occurs when a student has used someone else's work without acknowledging the original source. It is important to follow any guidance that you are provided with, and to ask for advice if you are uncertain how to refer to the literature you are using. Your university may use computer software to check for plagiarism. This facility may be offered to you to use as a formative tool to check your submission and correct any mistakes in referencing sources, or can be used by academic staff or the programme administrators to check a random sample of assignments.

TOP TIP

Listen to a podcast on plagiarism, or read the transcript provided on the following website. Although the information was not developed specifically for social work, the points they discuss are important in all academic programmes. You can listen to the views of both students and lecturers.

www.brookes.ac.uk/aske/resources.html Follow the links to 'Multimedia and other Resources'.

2.5.3 Confidentiality

It is important to protect the anonymity of individuals you may discuss within your work. This ensures individuals cannot be identified by readers of your assignment.

TOP TIP

- Make sure you explicitly state that confidentially has been adhered to.
- When anonymising your work, use an invented name rather than Mrs X, Mr Y or Child A to refer to service users and carers as it avoids dehumanising them.

2.5.4 Referencing

The purpose of referencing is to acknowledge the source of your information and ideas and to avoid plagiarising. References enable the reader to find the original source of your evidence should they wish to validate your argument. It is important for a reference to contain the author's name and date within text, and all subsequent publishing information at the end of your assignment. References also demonstrate to the reader the depth and breadth of your topic exploration, but remember quality, quantity and variety are equally important.

TOP TIP   Tips from students

- Don't lose marks by careless referencing. It's easy to leave this to the last task in an assignment, but rush it and you'll make the most elementary of errors. Reference as you go: that way you won't miss an author you've included in the text and not in the reference list and vice versa.
- There will be authors that you will regularly reference. Try working up a generic reference list of standard texts that you can copy and paste from. If you know those are correct you can really concentrate on getting those other journal or research references correct.
- Referencing takes many forms; ensure you read your university guidelines prior to completing an assignment and use the correct one for the programme. If in doubt seek support from lecturers, tutors, study skills groups or your subject librarian.
- Although your reference list is at the end of an assignment do be aware that the reader/ marker/assessor will often start here so do not underestimate its importance. A well-constructed reference list with a good range of relevant sources will give an indication of the potential quality of the assignment. Inadequate references indicate limited reading. It is essential to read a range of key sources for the subject and you will find pointers to what to read in the recommended reading list for that module.

2.6 USING ASSESSMENT FEEDBACK CONSTRUCTIVELY

Ideally, feedback will be timely, detailed and constructive and can be provided in a variety of formats.

Making use of the tutorial support available is highly recommended by the students we have worked with and learnt alongside. This support can take the form of individual or group sessions with your tutor. They may be included on the timetable as assignment workshops for specific modules or ones that provide generic assignment support. They can be an excellent starting point for assignment writing as they can enable you to explore ideas and tease out the salient points of a given subject. It is essential to utilise this support if you are struggling to understand a topic or to begin developing an assignment.

TOP TIP

Use your lecturers as valuable sources of information; do not be afraid to ask questions to enable them to share more of their subject knowledge and assessment experience with you.

The programme handbook will provide information about the processes and timings for handing in work and for return of the marked work. Feedback may take the form of typed feedback using a standard format, or a combination of generic class feedback and individual feedback; it may take the form of an audio file, or be provided both verbally and in typed format. You may experience peer feedback as part of a group activity where students award a proportion of the marks according to the efforts of all involved in a group assignment.

Receiving feedback, in whatever format, can be perceived as both worrying and exciting. You may have experienced negative criticisms of your coursework in the past, or you may feel anxious about failing. This type of belief can be extremely powerful. Having clear information about the principles of assessment and feedback can contribute to feeling more prepared, and we hope that by reading this chapter you will be able to approach feedback situations with more information and confidence.

It is important to read the feedback provided, not just look at the mark given, and to review your assignment in the light of the feedback to identify where you can improve. If you achieve a high mark, the feedback will reinforce the areas that you have done well in and signpost the areas for future development. If you have a low mark, the feedback should indicate the strengths of the assignment and also indicate clearly the areas for development in order to achieve a higher mark. If you receive a fail mark, the feedback should clearly set out what was missing, what worked well and what additional learning is needed in order to achieve a pass mark on resubmission. It is important to arrange a tutorial to discuss the assignment in detail and to develop a plan for resubmission, in line with the programme and university regulations.

The Assessment Standards Knowledge Exchange (ASKe undated a) at Oxford Brookes University recommends that markers provide overall feedback on what worked well and what needs to be improved, followed by specific feedback on the content of the assignment, in verbal and written form, with opportunities for questions.

Extracts from feedback: Example 1

You have demonstrated a passionate interest in this topic and have identified some important studies – from the classic work of Chris Jones to the more recent work of Stewart Collins. In places your sentence structure is complex and unclear and this detracts from the flow of the assignment as your points are sometimes difficult to follow. You have made very good use of your attendance at the regional social work conference though more on the national dimension would enhance the assignment and help you to meet the learning outcomes more fully. You have identified clearly the learning that you will be taking forward into your future practice.

Extracts from feedback: Example 2

I enjoyed reading this essay. You have produced a thoughtful assignment drawing on an area of practice familiar to you, whilst extending your skills and knowledge. You have made good use of the TAPUPA framework to analyse the material. The structure worked well and you showed a clear understanding of the research papers you identified. More on quantitative research would improve the assignment. Please ensure you capture the in-text references in your reference list – following the university referencing guide closely will help with this.

The above examples were provided for year 2 assignments which achieved marks within the 60–70 range. By considering areas of development such as structure and referencing the same students developed their academic writing skills and achieved first class marks in the remaining assignments.

Extracts from feedback: Example 3

Feedback from a placement observation undertaken by her Practice Educator.

The student was well prepared and had shared her planning notes and proposed objectives with me prior to the observation. Her preparation included identifying the correct forms required and reading the agency policy and procedure. The focus of the student's intervention shifted immediately before the start of the observation. The student was able to respond to the change and adapt her plans appropriately. After using ice breaking questions to relax and reassure the service user, the student agreed a plan for the observation with the service user. The student reminded the service user of my role and again sought her permission. I felt from the service user's response and body language that the student's enabling approach allowed the service user to feel that she had an active and valued role rather than just being a passive recipient. The student changed the pace of the interview according to the service user's needs. For example, at the beginning the service user expressed distress at a family upset. The student and service user agreed to discuss this first. The student could clearly see some of the service user's fixated views which were causing a degree of her distress. She was able to reflect-in-action, and used different tools to move forward the service user's thinking. The student closed the interview by (as at the beginning) returning to more general discussions and questions. The student then summarised what had taken place and how the service user now felt. The service user expressed her lessened anxiety and upset and thanked the student. The student checked all appropriate contact details were still available for the service user. They agreed a further appointment, which was planned for a date and time chosen by the service user.

You may have noted that the feedback is positive throughout and whilst the student was pleased about the feedback on her performance she wanted to have feedback on areas for development. This was achieved by discussing the feedback with the Practice Educator and drawing up an action plan to use in future Observations.

TOP TIP

Write a self-assessment action plan for future assignments to ensure you have assimilated and understood the feedback received. Over time look for patterns within the feedback and concentrate on these as areas you can develop with tutorial or peer support. By using this approach you are able to build on success rather than focus on supposed failure.

(ASKe undated b).

A LECTURER PERSPECTIVE

Feedback is also about 'feedforward' – providing comments on what worked well and what needs to be improved in order to build skills of assignment writing for future work, and for future social work practice.

I think carefully about the feedback, its purpose, the possible emotional content, the careful use of language, constructive and developmental, and not simply about specific errors in this particular assignment. Acknowledging the 'person' in the assignment can be important – particularly when marking reflective assignments. Students may feel personally attacked about their beliefs rather than the knowledge content. I aim to make feedback personal to that student, not just a list of commonly used feedback phrases, to assist the student in 'owning' the feedback in order to act on it in future.

What should you do after receiving feedback on your assignments? A constructive way forward is to make a clear plan to understand and act on the feedback. Overanalysing the feedback is not helpful, as for example there are not marks linked to each tick or comment provided.

CONCLUSION

We would like to share two sets of resources with you to enable you to consider the assessment developed by projects at two universities.

Firstly some advice to improve your assignments.

'Getting ready to start

- Read the assignment brief and look at the requirements and criteria. These are usually in your module guide.
- What does each criterion mean? If you're not sure, ask your tutor.
- Look at feedback you've received on previous assignments with similar criteria. Can you apply the advice to your current assignment?
- Are there examples of previously marked assignments? Judge the examples against the assessment criteria. Talk to others about what the criteria mean in practice, and what the expected standard is.

Working on your assignment

- Keep the assessment criteria nearby so that you know what's important.
- Find out if the module includes peer review sessions where you can talk to others about your draft work and how to improve it against each criterion.
- Use other resources available in the university to help you, e.g. referencing guides, peer assisted learning or upgrade sessions.
- Develop your self-assessment skills by trying to review and judge your work against the criteria.'

(ASKe project undated b)

This advice is built on in detail in the remaining chapters of this text.

Finally, we would like to share a list of 10 Principles of Assessment, developed by Liverpool John Moores University (2008, 7).

1. 'Assessment facilitates student learning and informs and supports student progress.
2. Assessment is an integral part of the course design process, appropriately aligned with learning outcomes.
3. Assessment must be inclusive and accessible.
4. There are clear and consistent assessment criteria.
5. Assessment is transparent.
6. Assessment is valid, reliable and free of bias.
7. Students have a responsibility to actively and honestly engage in the assessment process.
8. Students are provided with feedback on assessment which is timely, which promotes learning and facilitates improvement.
9. The management of assessment is efficient and effective, especially with regard to the amount and timings of assessment and staff and student workloads.
10. Assessment of students is underpinned by appropriate staff development.'

Now that you have learnt more about assessment and assignments you may wish to use the checklist to compare your experience of assessment. If you have any individual concerns about assessment then we recommend that you talk to your personal tutor or academic advisor in the first instance, and should there be shared concerns with other members of the class you may wish to involve your student programme representatives and approach the programme leader to attempt to resolve them positively.

We wish you good luck and effective and rewarding learning in your experiences of assessment!

CHAPTER 3
REFLECTION
AND REFLECTIVE
WRITING

This chapter will introduce you to the concept of reflection. By following the advice provided, and applying the techniques we demonstrate and using the tools we offer, you will become equipped to develop skills in reflection and reflective practice.

IN THIS CHAPTER WE WILL:

1 Consider what is reflection, how we do it and why we do it.
2 Consider how we might become reflective practitioners.
3 Describe some of the key models of reflection.
4 Consider possible teaching and learning activities involving reflective writing.
5 Introduce you to some possible assignment tasks associated with reflection.
6 Identify a range of tools and techniques for developing reflective practice and reflective writing.
7 Consider some of the barriers to becoming a reflective practitioner and offer tips for overcoming them.

We will be illustrating the points we are making with extracts from real assignments.

Warning: It is important that you do not copy these examples as this will constitute plagiarism, an academic offence. Remember, lecturers will be familiar with this chapter too!

The process of reflection enables social workers to integrate new perspectives and knowledge from a wide range of sources into their practice, in order to change, adapt and refine their practice depending on who they are working with and the context they are working in.

Being a reflective practitioner is one of the broad range of professional skills that are required of social work graduates. The Benchmarks for Social Work (QAA 2008 6.6) tell us that, by the end of their programme of study, social work graduates should be able to:

- reflect on and modify their behaviour in the light of experience;
- engage in a broad range of activities, including with other professionals and with service users and carers, to facilitate critical reflection. These include reading, self-directed study, research, a variety of forms of writing, lectures, discussion, seminars/tutorials, individual and group work, role-plays, presentations, projects, simulations and practice experience.

The Professional Capability Framework includes statements about skills of reflection in the domain of *Critical Reflection and Analysis*. For example, at entry to the programme you should be able to demonstrate

- 'an ability to reflect on and analyse own experience (educational, personal, formal and informal)'

and, at the stage of readiness for direct practice,

- 'understand the role of reflective practice and demonstrate basic skills of reflection'

and, at the end of the final placement,

- 'demonstrate a capacity for logical, systematic, critical and reflective reasoning and apply the theories and techniques of reflective practice' (College of Social Work 2012a).

However, reflection is not undertaken in isolation from other aspects of the social work role, and in order to acknowledge this it is embedded in all nine domains of the PCF: 'Critical reflection entails insight, exploratory and creative thinking for each unique piece of practice' (College of Social Work 2012b).

3.1 WHAT IS REFLECTION, HOW DO WE DO IT AND WHY DO WE DO IT?

A common misconception is that the process of reflection involves a process similar to simply looking in a mirror and describing what you see. We propose the analogy of looking in a muddy puddle to describe the process of reflection, with the use of tools and techniques to 'filter' the muddy puddle in order to make clearer sense of what you see. When looking at yourself in a puddle of water you will see an image which is constantly moving and changing. By using a critical lens to look more carefully and more deeply you begin the process of trying to filter this puddle, until you see yourself and your practice more clearly. The models and techniques we introduce you to will help to filter the information and bring it into a clearer focus.

Reflection involves not simply looking back at your practice or thought processes and describing them, as the notion of a mirror would suggest, but applying skills of analysis to what you did, why you did it, what knowledge, skills and values you drew on, and what you would do differently next time. You will also need to apply the critical thinking techniques discussed in Chapter 4 to help you move beyond description. Without employing a critical approach your written reflections may resemble a diary entry – containing a description of what you did and who said what. Reflection helps us to focus on the nuances of practice, on values and thought processes. However, to be able to develop reflective thinking or writing successfully requires practice. You may find this difficult at first, but please persevere as when you 'get it' it will intrinsically alter your thinking and future practice to the benefit of yourself, people you work with, and organisations you work for.

You must always take a questioning approach as a practitioner (we expand on this in Chapter 4). This includes questioning *your own* practice. The understanding gained by considering an event is then used to bring about change. Reflection is an essential tool of social work as it enables practitioners to appraise and respond to a situation with greater awareness of the influences brought by individuals and their wider social context. Reflective practice enables social workers to identify multiple perspectives and consider alternative explanations.

Another way of describing the process of reflection is *to think about what you did, why you did it and what this means for future practice.*

Lessons learnt when things go wrong on a day-to-day basis in practice (and in extreme cases which might have led to a public enquiry or serious case review) enables practitioners to re-evaluate judgements, understand better the processes involved and identify areas for development.

To summarise, reflection is the process of:

● attaching meaning to actions or events (why we did what we did);

● exploring emotional responses;

● developing a deeper understanding of yourself and the situation;

● transferring knowledge to future situations.

TAKE A MOMENT TO REFLECT...

If you are a current student on a social work degree programme think about the first few days at university and note down your recollections. (If you are reading this in preparation for university you might consider the first few days of starting a new job.)

● How did you interact with other students and the staff?

● What impressions did you take away with you?

● What were these impressions based on?

● How did you feel?

● How did you prepare for learning in the subjects you were introduced to (or the tasks involved in carrying out the job)?

● What could you have done differently?

● Have your first impressions changed over time? What caused them to change?

● What did you learn about yourself and others that will lead to you doing things differently?

Clearly we can't comment on the content of your answers but by thinking about these questions and responding you have been practising reflection. You may want to incorporate your responses to these questions into your learning journal if you are keeping one. We anticipate that your responses included at least some of the points in the summary above, that you have begun to see more clearly what influenced your experiences of the first few weeks of term, your feelings about what happened, that you have learnt about yourself and your approach to study and to new experiences and that you will use these insights during the rest of the course. (You may want to refer to the material in Chapter 1.)

Your responses to the activity are likely to involve the use of the word 'I'. This is referred to as writing 'in the first person' and whilst it is a feature of reflective writing it is not normally used in traditional academic essay writing. You will need to check the assignment guidelines carefully to establish which assignments, or sections of assignments, should be written in the 'first person' and which should not be.

3.2 HOW DO WE BECOME REFLECTIVE PRACTITIONERS?

What does it mean to *'reflect on and modify [your] behaviour in the light of experience'* (QAA 2008). It involves looking back on, weighing up, considering, pondering, reviewing *your* thoughts, feelings, actions and interactions. It is a technique used to review and re-process your ideas, feelings and actions in order to learn from them and refine them. Reflection is an important part of learning to be a social worker, of practising as a social worker and is one of the cornerstones of continuous professional development.

You are at the beginning phase of this, and as a social work student are measured against national academic criteria to ensure your readiness for post-qualifying practice. For instance, becoming a reflective practitioner involves 'a process in which a student reflects critically and evaluatively on past experience, recent performance, and feedback, and applies this information to the process of integrating awareness (including awareness of the impact of self on others) and new understanding, leading to improved performance' (QAA 2008).

As you are already discovering, becoming a social worker takes more than an acquisition of a set of knowledge, skills and values. Social workers need to be adept at flexibly responding to both expected and unexpected aspects of people and situations. This is achieved in part through reflective practice. Becoming a reflective practitioner is not simply about learning what reflection is and learning the vocabulary associated with it. It involves a life-long commitment to examine yourself and your practice and to apply the insights in order to continually adapt and develop your practice. Developing skills of reflective practice is not only a focus of social work education but is also a central part of other professions, in particular health professions and education. Some of our colleagues at Bournemouth University have contributed to this literature (Moon 2004, Rutter and Williams 2007, and Brown and Rutter 2008).

The QAA Benchmarks (2008: 4.7) tell us that:

'honours degree programmes in social work should be designed to help students learn to become accountable, *reflective*, critical and evaluative. This involves learning to:

- think critically about the complex social, legal, economic, political and cultural contexts in which social work practice is located

- work in a transparent and responsible way, balancing autonomy with complex, multiple and sometimes contradictory accountabilities (for example, to different service users, employing agencies, professional bodies and the wider society)

- exercise authority within complex frameworks of accountability and ethical and legal boundaries

- acquire and apply the habits of critical reflection, self-evaluation and consultation, and make appropriate use of research in decision-making about practice and in the evaluation of outcomes'. (Emphasis added)

It seems complicated; however, there are many ways of making sense of reflection and once you understand it from whatever perspective, you can begin to utilise it in your thinking and writing. Look at some examples of how reflection is understood:

3.2.1 What have students said about reflection?

In a study by Dempsey et al. (2001: 640) students reported that

reflective learning has been an essential tool in the processing of my learning during the year, but particularly while on placement. I found that I could take more from my experiences and identify some positive and negative aspects of the way that I work. Thus these were either reinforced or I began the process of changing. It has been invaluable.

You may be unsure about engaging in reflective learning, being unclear about the process and about the potential impact on your confidence. It is not unusual to feel de-skilled initially, or to be overcritical of your skills.

Take encouragement from another student in this study who said:

reflective learning has been new to me. It was uncomfortable at times, looking back at how you did things, why you did them and what you take away from it. It has also been challenging to engage in it, partly because it is new, but also because it creates space to question things – like your values, beliefs and attitudes. It above all has been a refreshing approach and very helpful tool in my learning throughout the year.

HOW DO OTHER WRITERS EXPLAIN REFLECTION?

Boud (1993) explains reflection as learning from experiences, that looking back on an experience or feeling enables individuals to understand and learn.

Dempsey et al. (2001) refer us to the work of Seidal and Blythe (1996) who described reflection as involving looking backwards, forwards, outwards and inwards.

Martyn (2006) uses the analogy of a mirror, describing reflection as *a replica or distortion of the original*.

Gimenez (2007) states that reflection is being better prepared for the future through the process of learning from what you do.

An important source on reflection is the work of Jan Fook. Fook and Askeland (2007: 521) describe critical reflection as 'the identification of deep-seated assumptions … incorporating an understanding of personal experiences within social, cultural and structural contexts' but with the primary focus of critical reflection as 'professional growth and social change'. Critical reflection is a term used by Fook (2012) to explain the process of reflecting on structures and power relationships in order to understand and challenge them and to avoid perpetuating them wherever possible. Fook (2012) emphasises that *critical* reflection is important as it leads to a change in practice in order not to perpetuate power inequalities. She emphasises the potential of critical reflection to challenge and change taken-for-granted thinking, processes and arrangements by examining implicit and hidden assumptions. Critical reflection operates as a catalyst to develop practice that responds more relevantly and creatively to practice situations.

3.3 REFLECTIVE MODELS

As we have seen, reflection can be described as the thinking process involved in analysing and evaluating practice which produces new understandings of the way we think and operate. The concepts of self-awareness, values and skills are integral alongside external knowledge which provides a framework/context in which the reflection occurs.

3.3.1 Dewey

As early as 1933 Dewey identified reflection as *the process through which learning from experience takes place* – a process similar to problem solving, which constantly re-evaluates beliefs and assumptions in the light of changing information and experience. This fits well with the complex scenario of social work, when new information is presented as part of ongoing assessment and as a result of the changing circumstances of service users and carers.

3.3.2 Schon

An adult educationalist, Schon (1983, 1991, 1996) developed the work of Dewey and has become widely known for his writing on reflection, and coined the term *the reflective practitioner*. He developed ideas around two main types of reflection:

- Reflection on action.
- Reflection in action.

These two processes may sound similar but they are in fact two very different aspects of reflection. The first involves the individuals reflecting after an event. This may occur through a journal, blog, sketch book, mind maps, or other means of 'thinking things through'. Our advice is to try different techniques until you find the one that works for you. The second, reflecting in action, occurs at the time of the event. This often happens unconsciously. Schon proposes making this a conscious activity, for example changing an approach midway through a session with a service user when you recognise that even though the approach seemed appropriate prior to the session it may be ineffective when actually put into practice. Schon proposed that this model allows for the development of *practice wisdom, or artistry* that enables practitioners to seek answers in circumstances where there is uncertainty or conflict.

3.3.3 Kolb's model

Kolb (1984) explores reflection by setting out a cycle of learning which views life experience as critical for learning. Kolb (1993: 155) believed that 'learning is the process whereby knowledge is created through the transformation of experience'.

Kolb's cycle of learning suggests that knowledge develops from life experiences and their interaction with theory. He states that learning takes place in four stages and for complete learning to occur the cycle must be completed. According to Kolb you must look back at an activity critically, determine what was useful or important and then take this knowledge forward to your next experience. In this model learning occurs as a result of the thoughts and ideas created by reflecting on an experience. Kolb acknowledges that learning does not always take place in this orderly way, that it is a continuous and ongoing process that is never fully complete, and that there may be several cycles of learning overlapping at the same time.

Argyris (1999) has suggested that Kolb's model is too dependent on the individual as it frames reflection in terms of a lone activity. Reflection can be effective as part of a peer activity, a professional activity such as supervision in the workplace, and group support. Kolb's model could lead

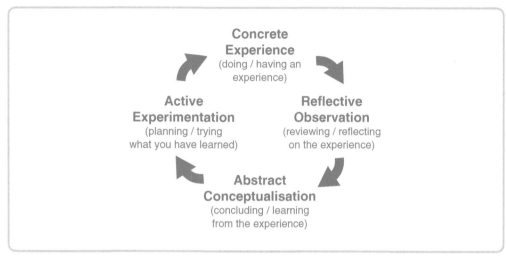

FIGURE 3.1 Kolb's model

Source: *Experiential Learning: Experience as the source of learning and development*, FT Prentice Hall (Kolb, D.A. 1984)

to an interpretation that the simple accumulation of learning automatically leads to more effective practice, where in reality learning is a dynamic and complex process.

CONSIDER AN EVENT IN YOUR LIFE AND RELATE THIS TO KOLB'S CYCLE OF LEARNING

- What was the event, what happened?
- How and when did you reflect on it – during or after, or both?
- What did you learn?
- As a result, what did you do differently in the future?

Comment

By considering experiences in this way you will have already been using some of the skills of reflective practice that you will develop further during your social work studies.

3.3.4 Gibbs' model

Gibbs (1988) offers a model which breaks down reflection into a series of stages and questions. This model makes a clear link between reflection and social work practice as it explicitly asks about feelings as well as thoughts.

Description – What happened?

Feelings – What were you thinking and feeling?

Evaluation – What was good and bad about the experience?

Analysis – What sense can you make of the situation?

Conclusion – What else could you have done?

Action Plan – What was learnt? If it arose again, what would you do differently?

3.3.5 Gimenez

Gimenez (2007) offers a useful three-stage reflective cycle (see Figure 3.2) which comprehensively breaks down not only the stages but what analytical and evaluative skills transform a piece into critical reflection.

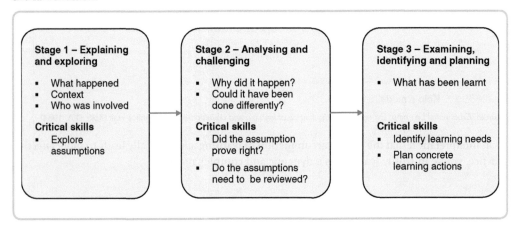

FIGURE 3.2 Three-stage reflective cycle (Adapted from Gimenez 2007).

3.4 POSSIBLE TEACHING AND LEARNING ACTIVITIES INVOLVING REFLECTIVE WRITING

3.4.1 Online group discussion to support reflection

Reflection on learning and on practice is not necessarily a dialogue, either spoken or written, between you and your lecturer or between you and your practice educator but may be part of group activities. On your course you are likely to have the opportunity to engage in both face-to-face and online group discussions designed to develop reflective skills in an interactive, collaborative and cooperative environment. Through a group approach students can learn from one another, test out and develop their understanding, develop greater awareness of their values and beliefs, challenge and be challenged in a supportive and safe learning environment.

You may initially find posting your reflections on an online discussion forum or blog daunting, compared to a more private approach of a written account seen only by the lecturer or practice educator, but it is important to persevere. A research-minded approach by a group of lecturers at an American university (Bye et al. 2009) who used both online group discussions and individual reflective learning activities found that students believed they had learnt more from the online discussions. We hope this will encourage you to engage with any web-based activities that are provided for you on your programme.

In a very different subject area, that of public relations, a study in Australia by Wolf (2010) into student experiences of using a reflective blog whilst on placement found encouraging results.

In an earlier social work study by Quinney (2005), long before the use of social media became widespread, social work students used a website to support learning in practice, including the use of a discussion forum. Students new to using technology gained confidence, with one student commenting that, despite concerns that using technology was daunting, 'you just click and type' (Quinney 2005: 447). Both Wolf's (2010) and Quinney's (2005) studies found that using a blog or discussion forum enabled students to feel 'connected' to one another whilst on placement.

3.4.2 Skills labs

You may have the opportunity to participate in skills lab activities which provide opportunities for reflective learning prior to or alongside undertaking direct practice in an agency setting. It is not unusual for these interactions to be filmed and replayed for reflective learning opportunities. Various approaches are used to undertake role-play of a face-to-face interview, with an actor, a fellow student, a member of the programme team, or a service user.

3.4.3 Group activities

You may be involved in a group activity or group project as part of the course. This might be with other social work students or with students from other disciplines. The assessed work may include a reflection on group processes and your contribution, performance and learning.

Here are some reflections from Sarah when engaged in an inter-professional group assignment task.

> I recognised that conflict and challenge was sometimes directed at individuals and experienced as personal attacks. I needed to examine my need to be liked and accepted in the group. I recall not wishing to be perceived as the leader, because group acceptance was my priority and my emotional well-being was as important as the success of the group project. I later realised that I was subconsciously seeking a position of power and influence and this seems to have become more important as I became more confident in the group. I now understand that not everything I do is consciously thought through and that my ability to operate as a team player is dependent, to some extent, on the team playing by my rules.

3.4.4 Reflection on critical incidents in placement

A common method of gathering evidence of your abilities to reflect on the transfer of learning in practice placements and your interventions with service users, carers, immediate colleagues and other professionals is the use of critical incident reports. An example of a format for this is provided later in this chapter, devised by Green Lister and Crisp (2007). However, your programme may use different templates and tools.

3.4.5 What does reflective writing look like?

Recording your reflections on paper, or typing them, may initially seem challenging. However, it is a vital part of reflection as the process supports and develops reflective and critical thinking. Brown and Rutter (2008) liken writing skills to thinking skills, suggesting that they are fundamentally the same. They suggest that because writing is slower than thinking it allows us to achieve more in terms of exploring and understanding the connections of past experience and current practice. This they suggest enables us to gain an understanding of different perspectives.

Reflective writing is not simply an opportunity to describe an event. It is an opportunity to demonstrate that you review your practice and learn from it. As a rule reflective writing should demonstrate an understanding, and application, of theory, values and practice skills. It should demonstrate developmental milestones within your practice and clearly identify learning outcomes. This requires reflecting on how you used social work skills, challenged assumptions and judgements, utilised social work values and adhered to the principles of anti-oppressive practice. You might find it helpful to ask yourself the following questions before you begin writing, to promote a reflective approach.

- What did you think, why did you think this and what was the impact?
- How did you feel and how did you use these feelings?
- How have you been socially constructed/shaped by your environment to view the situation?
- What impact might this have had?
- How did the differences between you and the people you are working with (service users and other professionals) impact on your practice?
- How did you communicate, why did you communicate in this way, what was the impact?
- What skills did you use, how did you use them, what was the impact?
- What research/knowledge did you draw on? What do you need to learn more about?
- What went well/what went badly and why?
- Did you change approach at any stage, if so why and what was the impact?
- Have you drawn on and referred to social work literature?

One argument for enjoying reflective writing is that it helps you to take ownership of your assignments. Engaging in reflection helps you to better understand social behaviour, your own practice and thought processes.

You may find the use of 'I' in reflective writing takes practice. Used well, this personal style gives a feeling of personal reflection that is not normally present in traditional academic writing. Writing in the first person enables greater exploration of you as an individual. It offers the opportunity to critique your own practice and demonstrate an increased level of self-awareness. However, this style of writing can result in a descriptive and narrative account of *I did this* and *then I did that*, which should as a rule be avoided.

It is important to support what you are saying with academic literature. This may appear confusing and contradictory as on the one hand we are saying you should write in the first person, and then on the other we are saying use published work to support your reflection. Think of it like this. If you use (which you should) knowledge and research gained from published work to support and frame your practice, you should equally use it to support and frame reflection. Without utilising recognised published work your reflective writing will appear as anecdotal only. You must validate and support your claim to knowledge through the use of references.

The people marking your assignments will read your work through a critical lens. It is useful to bear this in mind in order to pre-empt questions such as:

- What does this mean for social work practice?
- How have you drawn this conclusion?
- What evidence is there to support this?

By ensuring you have provided explanation and evidence from the literature, you are adding greater transparency to your work. In addition, as a qualified social worker you will be expected by colleagues, managers and service users to be able to justify your decisions. Engaging in reflection enables you to begin to develop these skills and is therefore fundamental to your social work development. Through developing these skills during the social work course you are following you will become more confident to apply them when you qualify.

Counter-arguments are a useful technique to employ in your writing and can be powerful; by introducing them into your reflective assignments you are demonstrating that you have considered other perspectives, have applied a critical perspective to your reflection, and have understood the literature that supports it. By introducing counter-arguments you can begin to clarify and sharpen your ideas and learning and to apply a critical perspective to what you are thinking and writing.

You may be tempted to include as much information as possible in your reflective writing. The risk here is that you may lose the depth of thinking. Try to analyse only the main points by picking out the key values, skills, legislation and theories. When reflecting, the smallest of incidents can lead to a wealth of reflection. 'Focussing down' in this way gives you the space and time to really consider and comment on issues from a range of perspectives. You will see examples of what we mean below, when we use extracts from student assignments to illustrate different aspects of reflective writing. These are illustrations of how some students have approached reflective writing, and are not intended as a definitive guide.

We will now look more closely at how to evidence critical reflection. The table on p. 46 offers a useful checklist for writing reflectively.

3.4.6 Integrating social work values into reflective writing

Values are a set of overarching principles that social workers must espouse in order to promote social change, social justice and maintain an empowering approach to their practice (BASW 2012, College of Social Work 2012 a). A central component of anti-oppressive practice is a social worker's awareness of their values. Values, therefore, should be a central theme running through any reflective work you may produce. However, as Shardlow (2002: 30) so graphically and memorably describes, this can be complex even for the most reflective individuals. He states that

> Getting to grips with social work values and ethics is rather like picking up a live, large fish out of a running stream. Even if you are lucky enough to grab a fish, the chances are that just when you think you have caught it, the fish will vigorously slither out of your hands and jump back into the stream.

His statement captures how complex and challenging it can be to recognise and adhere to our values. Values should normally be a constant point of discussion throughout reflective assignments. There should be recognition of their fundamental role within your practice. You should demonstrate that you understand and can use values to ensure that concepts such as citizenship and participation are promoted, as well as referring to concepts such as oppression and segregation. It is important to check the assignment guidelines carefully to establish how you are expected to refer to social work values in your written work.

WHAT?   Your reflections

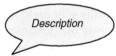

Description

- What did you do?
- What happened?
- What did you feel?

HOW?

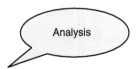

Analysis

- How did you do it?
- What made you choose that approach?
- Why not another method?
- What was your aim?

Include what theory/research/experiences/values influenced your action.
Consider the assumptions that informed your judgements.
How did you feel?
Reflect on what you thought and felt before, during and after the intervention/interaction.

WEIGH UP

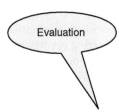

Evaluation

- To what extent your goals were met.
- The impact of other factors.
- The strengths and weaknesses of your action.

Consider the wider context of influence and how the situation could be viewed from an alternative perspective.

WHAT NEXT?

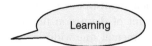

Learning

- What does this mean for your future practice?
- What does this mean for people you work with?
- How has this changed your beliefs or led to alternative insights? What are your future development needs?
- Have you been inspired to research further in any particular area?

(Adapted from Brown and Rutter 2008)

It is useful to acknowledge and discuss any ethical dilemmas you may have faced. These could be instructions from other staff in placements which are not congruent with social work values, or how social work values do not always sit comfortably with particular pieces of legislation. For example, the Mental Health Act 1983 could be interpreted as oppressive in parts, particularly in the powers to detain people in hospital on the grounds of apparent mental instability. A debate about ethical dilemmas such as the issue of care versus control would highlight the challenge of anti-oppressive practice.

Values can operate at a conscious or subconscious level. We do not have to be openly aware of our values for them to influence our actions and the decisions we make. However, with greater awareness comes an increased ability to ensure our actions are congruent with the values we recognise as important. It is through the process of reflection that we can improve our awareness. This can enable us to both recognise aspects of our practice that we were unaware of at the time, and recognise the need for development, ensuring our future practice adheres to the fundamental principles which underpin effective social work practice.

Sometimes students are reluctant to acknowledge non-adherence to social work values. They may refer to areas or incidences of poor practice in general, but do not explicitly link this to their action, their value base or their developmental needs. They may be concerned that they might be judged as demonstrating poor practice. However, by acknowledging areas in need of development, and explicitly highlighting these, the student is demonstrating that their practice is guided by sound values, and through reflection they are able to challenge and adapt.

A final point on this subject is offered by Preston-Shoot (1996: 31). He states that 'values are only as good as the actions they prompt'.

It is important not only to be intellectually committed to social work values but also to be able to demonstrate how you have applied them. When reflecting on your use of values, make clear, conscious and explicit links between the value statement in discussion and the actual aspect of your practice you are reflecting on. There are several publications that explore values in the context of social work, including Banks (2012) and Parrott (2006), and you are likely to have been provided with recommendations for specific reading on this important topic.

3.5 ASSIGNMENTS

We will use extracts from actual assignments to illustrate the range of styles of reflective writing.

Assignment extract 1

A student's first attempt to write reflectively, early in the first placement.

I reflected on my early feelings about our interactions by considering my initial impression of Miss B. Swearing seemed a normal part of her language and she appeared defensive and verbally aggressive. I considered whether my feelings were influenced through stereotypes and current media interest, and realised that my knowledge of young offenders with drug issues was influenced by media perspectives. I was also aware of a number of differences between Miss B and myself that impacted upon our relationship and balance of power, the greater of which were our diverse life experiences. Miss B's experience of drugs and prostitution, which formed the greater part of her teenage and adult life, indicated she belonged to a culture that I had little knowledge of. Her losses including the removal of her daughter negatively influenced her perception of herself and the value of relationships. However, as our relationship developed, I also recognised some similarities in terms of our life experiences, such as becoming a young parent. Being aware of professional boundaries meant that I was unable to share this common ground with Miss B, but it gave me some empathy and insight into her life chances, and enabled me to demonstrate positive unconditional regard. Over time, I became aware of my assumptions and stereotypical beliefs and recognised that I needed to gain further knowledge about this client group to minimise the risk of stereotyping. I also need to learn greater skills in risk assessment to ensure I make informed judgements rather than being judgemental. This is a skill that would have made my initial relationship with Miss B more professional and consequently more useful. When starting a new relationship with any service user in the future I will ensure that these learning needs are at the forefront of my mind to enable me to reflect 'in' practice as well as reflecting 'on' my practice.

Lecturer commentary

In this extract the student demonstrates growing self-awareness and reflects on what she might do differently. Attention is drawn to concepts including power, risk and loss, demonstrating insight into the complexity of the service user's situation. An area for development is the use of specific references to literature to illustrate the points being made.

3.5.1 Integrating issues of diversity/power/anti-oppressive practice/self-identity into reflective writing

The evident and hidden differences between people, for example in terms of their gender, race, political allegiances, sexuality, or age will undoubtedly impact on the way we interact, both professionally and personally. It is for this reason that social workers require an acute awareness of their own beliefs, coupled with an understanding of their origins and of the power dynamics that may exist between them and the service users they are working with. By acknowledging who *you* are, where your beliefs originated and how this will impact on service users, you will be able to evidence that you are actively attempting to practise anti-oppressively.

Assignment extract 2

Reflecting on completing a person-centred plan (PCP) with Sam, a service user with learning disabilities. The student had been informed by staff that Sam could not read or write.

About 10 minutes into completing his PCP, Sam asked if he could write his own plan rather than me doing it for him. At this stage it became apparent that the information I had received about Sam's literacy ability was inaccurate (an example of reflection in action). I considered whether this might be based on assumptions about the limited ability of people with learning disabilities. Until this point I had viewed myself as a student who has a good understanding of his own value base, and that I adhere to this at all times. However, the process of reflection has enabled me to see that I too held stereotypes of this service user group, which is why I did not question staff when they said Sam could not read or write, neither did I talk to Sam first to find out how he wanted the session structured. This is clear evidence that I was not practising fully in accordance with social work values. This would have contributed to an oppressive form of practice, which Dowling et al. (2007) suggest maintains a focus on disability. By not establishing Sam's abilities at the start of the session, I disempowered him by removing ownership of his plan and taking control of the session. Dowling et al. (2007) suggest that focussing on his disability and not his abilities would have led me to limit his options for development and ownership.

Dowling et al. (2007) suggest PCP requires professionals to surrender power and control over someone's life. I thought that by completing the writing portion of the plan the session was more productive and the plan would be clearer and more precise, removing pressure from Sam. However, Sam's assertiveness alerted me to how controlling I may have been. Realising this, I changed my approach, situating him as expert, through the use of the Exchange Model (Smales et al. 1994, cited Milner and O'Byrne 2002). Responding to Sam's request to write his own plan appeared to empower him; he almost instantly appeared to place greater trust in me which enabled a free flow of information, which was further enhanced by my use of both open and closed questions. By adapting my approach and enabling Sam to have greater control, I was able to conclude the session positively, whilst being confident that after a bad beginning I had on the whole practised in an anti-oppressive manner whilst adhering to fundamental values such as individualisation and client self-determination. However, I have also gained an increased awareness of how stereotypes can impact on my adherence to social work values, having a negative impact on the service users I work with.

Lecturer commentary

In this piece of reflective writing the student engages in *critical* reflection (Fook 2012), drawing attention to power imbalances and the potentially oppressive practice as a result of not being confident, experienced or assertive enough to question initially. By engaging in reflection *in* action the student quickly recognised the misinformation and adjusted his practice. He reflects openly and honestly about the situation he has found himself in and identifies learning and implications for future practice. He refers to values, anti-oppressive practice, and power relationships.

This extract has demonstrated how to

- use both positive and negative examples;
- be specific and explicit;
- do things differently in the future and identify the learning points;
- be concise – you will have used a range of values, pick the most pertinent ones and discuss them (unless you have been given different guidance in the assignment guidelines);
- reinforce the points you are making with reference to published authors;
- synthesise several themes.

Assignment extract 3

Reflecting on identity and self-awareness

When I began to write reflectively, lecturers would write on my assignment 'but who are *you*?'. Initially I was puzzled as they had my name on the front sheet. Later, I realised that 'who are you' referred to my age, gender, life experiences and its impact on my practice. Later still, I began to understand that to critically reflect is to look beyond the surface interactions and analyse both myself and the service user's position within society. From this point I could reflect on my inter-actions in light of who I am and who the service user was. I had talked about who the service user was but had neglected to acknowledge who I was and the impact of this on the interaction. Finally, I was able to reflect on the above, recognising that my position within society would have created an imbalance of power between myself and the service users. This enabled more robust and insightful reflections that interweaved the service user, myself, our impact on each other and the impact of power on our relationship. As my skills grew, I began to appreciate the value of self-awareness in terms of the insight this gave into mine and others' unique frames of reference. It took a while for me to understand and begin to reflect on this.

We have provided a simple yet effective table to ensure you consider areas of difference between yourself and the service users you are working with to promote self-awareness.

What is your	What is the service user's	How might this influence the interaction?
Gender	**Gender**	
Age	Age	
Ethnicity	Ethnicity	
Culture	Culture	
Educational background	Educational background	
Perception of class (how do you view yourself?)	Perception of class (how do you view yourself?)	
Religion	Religion	

3.5.2 Why should critical reflection involve an awareness of power and diversity?

During the social work degree you are likely to consider important questions such as 'what is social work for?' You will need to consider whether social workers are agents of social control or social change; agents of the state or an autonomous profession seeking to empower and create positive changes in people's lives. These questions will be the focal point of many learning sessions throughout your degree. The concept of anti-oppressive practice is fundamental if social workers are to work towards a model of social work which promotes social justice, whilst challenging oppressive structures and social relationships. Healy (2005) reminds us that, like other modern forms of critical practice, anti-oppressive practice draws on the debate from other types of critical social work (anti-discriminatory, anti-racist and black perspectives, structural social work, feminism). She states that it emphasises:

- the structural origins of service users' problems;
- an orientation towards radical social change;
- a critical analysis of practice relations and an attempt to transform these relationships in practice.

It is important to recognise that practitioners can unconsciously add to oppressive structures and relationships. The extract below is an example of how we can behave oppressively if consideration is not given to our own identity and how this interacts with the identity of others.

Assignment extract 4

Example of white, 24-year-old, middle class student reflecting on being an anti-racist practitioner

Arguably viewing my ethnicity as a 'non-issue' has had an impact on my practice. It is clear throughout this placement that I demonstrated an approach which Dominelli (1997) describes as the colour blind approach. I had prided myself on treating everyone the same; this included the one black service user present. I thought the purpose of anti-racist practice was to treat everyone equally no matter what their skin colour. Reflection has enabled me to see that this naïve view, as Dominelli (1997) argued, led me to reduce everyone to the same common denominator without regard to the position they actually occupy either as an individual or as a member of a social group.

This colour blind approach arose from my inability to see the power I possessed through my skin colour, and the consequent lack of power experienced by ethnic minority groups. Reflection has stirred strong emotions of guilt, feelings of ignorance and anger at myself, as Dominelli (1997) argues this approach contains aspects which endorse white supremacy. Tatum (1994) suggests that white students learning about racism experience feelings similar to my own and this, she suggests, leads many to resist learning. Applying the knowledge I gained from reading academic texts and reflecting on my practice enabled me to acknowledge my oppressive ways however painful this was and to change my practice as a result.

Lecturer commentary

In this extract the student has reflected on some uncomfortable aspects of learning. Social work education and training can be unsettling and disruptive when beliefs are challenged and new ways of viewing 'the world' are developing. The social work degree can be emotionally demanding and it is important to develop strong support networks, and to make use of support services provided by the university.

TOP TIP — Points to consider in reflective writing

- Be explicit about your thoughts and feelings.
- Acknowledge oppressive practice, whilst stating how you have recognised it and plan to change.
- Make explicit reference to your own identity and how this influenced your practice.
- Make it personal to you by referring to the merits of adopting anti-oppressive practice, and saying how this impacts on service users.
- Consider your social influences, upbringing, gender, sexuality and how these might impact on your practice.

- If you considered issues of diversity prior to the interaction, how did you accommodate this into your practice, and if not how did this affect your practice?

- Did you think you were well prepared but later, on reflection, found that you had missed something, did this have an impact?

- Have you evaluated your practice in relation to power structures, including oppression and discrimination as a result of, for example, sexism, racism and ageism?

You need to demonstrate clearly that you have considered these issues. You may want to discuss the complexity of the power between you and the service users you are reflecting on. For example, some find it problematical to assess who actually holds the greater power in the client–social worker relationship. This is not always as obvious as many believe, as the service user can belong to both powerful and less powerful groups simultaneously. They could for example be from the more powerful or dominant gender group, but be disempowered through a disability. As a social work student, you could belong to multiple oppressed groups, if you were black, female, disabled and from a working class background. However, you hold power as a result of your professional status, albeit as a student. The service user may demonstrate power through aggressive or angry behaviour and it is important to remain calm and assertive. Issues of diversity and power influence how we act in many different environments, including how we receive and give information, how we build relationships and how we view the world.

Fook (2012) insightfully highlights that people do not easily fit into 'powerful' or 'powerless' groupings, sometimes having membership of both at the same time. Also, members of powerless groups do not necessarily agree on the form of their empowerment. She goes on to say that some people may find an experience empowering where others find the same experience disempowering. To practise anti-oppressively is to acknowledge this at the onset of your work. It is to clearly indicate within text that you have opened up the communication channels and let the service user lead any discussions or interventions. You should make explicit reference to the diversity and power differences between you and the service user, and how you accommodated this within your practice. Or how your identity made you think or act in a certain way. Always remember to evaluate how this may have had an impact on the service user (see Extract 2).

3.5.3 Integrating theories into reflective writing

Social work theories can be used to predict a situation, understand it, or guide us through appropriate interventions. Utilising a variety of social work theories is therefore crucial for effective social work practice. Reflective writing provides the opportunity to demonstrate that you have developed a working knowledge of the application of these theories. However, many students struggle to convey this concisely within their text.

Example 1

I have found implementing Thompson's PCS model exciting yet challenging in equal measures. It has allowed me to highlight many oppressive views I subconsciously harboured. I now recognise that my views further enhanced the structural oppression felt by many. This in turn has enabled me to adapt my practice so I am working anti-oppressively, and in keeping with my social work value base. This has opened up possibilities for my practice to develop.

Example 2

Thompson's PCS model enables practitioners to look at micro level and macro level interactions. It offers an exciting theoretic basis to recognise that discrimination operates at three separate levels, the personal, cultural and structural levels of society. Utilising this theory can enable practitioners to open up the possibility of developing their practice through recognition of oppression and discrimination.

The first passage, Example 1, is written in 'the first person' and gives the impression that the student has actively engaged with Thompson's model and is actively using it in their practice. The second paragraph is more appropriate to non-reflective writing, and feels disengaged from practice. It does not convey any emotion, or 'use of self' and does not give the impression that the student actively uses this model in their practice. It demonstrates only a minimal awareness of what the theory could do if applied, whereas the first passage clearly states the impact on the student's practice.

Theories can be modified through practice and be adapted and created during practice. The two processes often occur simultaneously, as we make sense of the situations we encounter. The process of reflection enables us to acknowledge what theories, values and skills we have drawn on, and to evaluate their effectiveness.

Consider linking theories to anti-oppressive practice, values and frameworks to demonstrate your increased understanding and development.

- Use published work to back up your argument and relate it directly to your practice.
- Do not attempt to discuss every theory you may have used – it is important to demonstrate depth of thinking, not simply breadth of ideas.

Assignment extract 5

In this example a final year student reflects on using social work theories to develop an understanding of the possible oppression a service user, Geoff, may have experienced.

Foucault (1965, cited Haralambos et al. 2000) suggests that any signs of irrational behaviour have come to be defined as madness, and people exhibiting these signs will be confined, controlled and contained in isolation like lepers away from mainstream society. He alludes to what he calls the 'medical gaze', which he argues allows for the constant surveillance and monitoring of individuals like Geoff, by turning all 'deviants' into medical subjects.

Goffman (1968, cited Haralambos et al. 2000) argues that the labels imposed by psychiatry will only be applied by individuals who have something to gain from its application, and once applied the person's self-image is taken away and they are expected to conform to institutional rules. Geoff's experiences mirror many of Goffman's points, as at times he failed to follow the rules imposed by his 'capturers', which according to his notes was further evidence of mental illness, and a greater need for him to be detained and managed. Geoff has spoken of wanting to be treated as an individual with respect and dignity, this was seen as a sign of him exhibiting symptoms and lacking insight. However, Hamilton and Roper (2006) would surmise that Geoff was in fact correctly analysing his status within the system. This they suggest is an insidious form of oppression that appears like compassion, with the removal of Geoff's rights in the interest of his well-being. Even though Geoff had two yearly tribunal hearings to discuss discharge, he had no resisting position, due to the power imbalance between him and the professionals. Hamilton and

Roper (2006) highlight this power imbalance effectively in terms of playing games. They surmise that he cannot say I am feeling mentally well, as this may be evidence that he is in fact unwell. In this construction, true insight is unachievable, as one way or another the characterisation has to be given through the mechanisms of psychiatry.

Applying the central assumption of social constructionism whilst utilising a Foucauldian ideology has enabled me to view my previous thoughts on Geoff as oppressive, and has highlighted the further oppression he may have experienced over the last 30 years. It enabled me to see that Geoff's identity itself could have been socially constructed by psychiatry, consequently making his deviance easier to control. This is a pertinent point if you consider that Geoff had no diagnosed mental illness and only a borderline learning disability prior to being detained under the Mental Health Act (1983). Consequently, this improved my ability to apply social work values and those set out in the NIMHE framework (2004). I will demonstrate how I adopted this increased understanding into practice later in this assignment, for now I will continue to focus on developing a creative insight into my own practice and the oppression Geoff may have experienced.

Lecturer commentary

The extract demonstrates very able use of literature and theories derived from sociology. However, this style of writing does not capture the 'use of self' and personal insights that are a distinct quality of reflective writing. It contains many of the features of critical thinking and critical writing that are the focus of Chapter 4.

3.5.4 Integrating awareness of social work skills into reflective writing

Thompson (2000) provides an overview of what he describes as the basis social work skills; however, he humorously, suggests that one would require an encyclopaedia to detail all the skills a social worker can potentially utilise. Thompson includes the following:

- Communication skills
- Self-awareness skills
- Analytical skills
- An ability to handle feelings
- Self-management skills
- Presentation skills
- Co-ordination skills
- Sensitivity and observational skills
- Refection skills
- Creativity
- Thinking on your feet
- Humility
- Resilience
- Partnership skills
- Survival skills.

Depending on your previous experience and learning during the course you may already possess some of these skills, and they will continue to develop during the social work course you are following. A useful exercise is to construct a skills development plan, in which you highlight areas of strengths and weaknesses and consider how you intend to develop them. When writing reflective accounts it is important to consider the skills used and the extent of your mastery of them.

Assignment extract 6

A social work student's reflections, in her final placement, on planning to meet with another professional who had been working with Anna, a 14-year-old service user.

It transpired that the counsellor had given Anna her personal mobile number and befriended her on a social network site thus fuelling Anna's need for love and attention. I considered that this relationship had to be challenged as I felt it had crossed the boundaries of professionalism and furthermore was not helping Anna engage with support from more appropriate sources. Knowing this did not make my challenge to this situation easier. I found I struggled to separate my regard for a fellow professional from what I believed was damaging practice. I discussed the situation with my team leader and Practice Educator in order to be very clear in my mind as to the potential damage this could cause Anna and to ensure I did not further collude or ignore the boundary issues. I also felt worried about the conversation I would have, in terms of the counsellor's possible responses to me. I thought carefully about what I would say, how I would say it, and what my tone and pace of voice and other non-verbal cues would communicate to the counsellor. When reflecting on this I realised my concern over other people's opinions of me as 'just a student' had been a hidden factor in my fear of challenging. In future practice, the learning from this experience and my wider reading has helped me to feel more confident to challenge the work of other professionals where I am concerned about the impact of their actions on young people.

Lecturer's comment

This reflective account demonstrates the importance of developing assertiveness skills, and the value of preparation and seeking advice and support from the team leader and practice educator. High quality supervision is essential, as is learning from other colleagues.

'Supervision should be open and supportive focussing on the quality of decisions, good risk analysis and improving the outcomes for children.'

(Laming 2009: 32)

When considering what to focus on in a reflective account it is important to be aware that the smallest of incidents can lead to a wealth of reflection. Focussing down gives you the opportunity to fully consider and comment on issues from a range of perspectives. The account would be strengthened with reference to appropriate literature.

3.5.5 Integrating the identification of future learning needs

The following reflective extract is used to demonstrate that reflective writing is not always undertaken in response to practice scenarios but can form part of professional and personal development planning by reviewing learning and goal setting.

Assignment extract 7

A student reflecting on their learning and personal development needs on completing their first placement.

My awareness has increased with regard to the stereotypes and assumptions which I unconsciously harbour, and the impact these have on others. I recognise the importance of considering the origins of my beliefs and exploring how they became an inherent aspect of my world view. When considering my need to 'please' and be 'liked', using processes including Transactional Analysis, I now recognise that my confidence in practice settings is sometimes low and I often view others as better than me. In addition, when feeling threatened I can make decisions based on the view of other professionals rather than in the best interest of the service user. This could not only affect my ability to manage the service user's risks, but my ability to assess and advocate for service users. The knowledge gained through reflection has been essential in terms of my practice development. It has heightened awareness of my personal development needs, and provides insight into weaker areas of practice which can be explored further through reflective supervision and peer feedback. With this increased awareness/confidence I can adapt my future practice to be more flexible to the needs of the service users I interact with. I believe the skill gained from this reflection will enable me to react much quicker, and seek support at a much early stage.

Assignment extract 8

An extract from an assignment in which students were required to reflect on their learning about the value of research to inform practice.

Reflecting on my learning has enabled me to explore what knowledge, experience and feelings I had about using research to inform my practice, and challenge my preconceived assumptions. I have previously approached research papers with considerable trepidation, not least because I felt my lack of knowledge about research terminology would prevent me from understanding them fully. I considered my practice to be evidence based, however this assignment has enabled me to understand where my knowledge has been reliant on evidence disseminated by the organisation, or easier reading texts rather than a wide range of more robust sources of 'evidence'. My new skills of research-mindedness have stimulated an enthusiasm for research. As a seconded student my increased skills and knowledge will enable me to immediately share my new knowledge within my team, providing the opportunity to reconsider some of our practice.

3.5.6 Comment

In the concluding part of an assignment for a research awareness module, students were asked to reflect on their learning, changing from the '3rd person' to the '1st person' in writing style. Identifying learning and its value for future practice was an integral part of the assignment, demonstrating not only knowledge of research-mindedness but also a commitment to using this to make a difference in practice.

3.6 TOOLS AND TECHNIQUES TO AID REFLECTION

3.6.1 Tool 1

The Critical Incident Analysis Framework (Green Lister and Crisp 2007)

The framework, consisting of five sets of questions, was tested by students at the University of Glasgow undertaking their second practice-learning placement, and the experience of the student and practice educator of using this formed part of a larger research project. This particular framework is designed to be applied to commonplace or significant events.

A student who was interviewed about the use of the Framework commented: 'It clarified what is meant by reflection and analysis and helped me consolidate what I thought. It is logical and structured.' (Green Lister and Crisp 2007: 51)

Their small-scale research project into the use of the framework indicated that the students reported benefits that included the following:

- it provided a clear structure;
- it supported the integration of theory to practice;
- it provided the opportunity to focus on values and the emotional impact of exploring values.

If you would like to use this Framework to help you reflect on your practice, use the headings set out here. For full details of the framework, you will need to access the peer-reviewed journal article (Green Lister and Crisp 2007) in which it appears. (Please note that the journal it is published in is now called *Practice; Social Work in Action*. See *Further reading* at the end of this chapter.)

CRITICAL INCIDENT FRAMEWORK

1. Account of the incident
2. Initial responses to the incident
3. Issues and dilemmas highlighted by this incident
4. Learning
5. Outcomes

3.6.2 Tool 2

The DEAL model, which stands for Describe, Examine, and Articulate Learning

Lay and McGuire (2010), for structured critical reflection. This is a model developed for social work from the work of Ash et al. (2006) at the Indiana School of Social Work, in Illinois, USA, and is part of an ongoing evaluation as part of research-minded approach to learning and teaching. (To read the full article please see *Further reading* at the end of this chapter.)

Step 1

Describe (in fair detail, the who, why, what, where and when as objectively as possible) the experience, the activity or the reading related to course objectives. Think about a class discussion, lecture, reading, and focus on what stood out for you as a learning experience. Be sure to cite sources.

Step 2

Examine, in accordance with the course learning objectives and past, current and potential life experience (e.g. personal, practice placement, employment) a specific concept, theory or issue. The goal is to examine and integrate. Remember to cite sources.

Step 3

Articulate learning

- What did I learn?
- How did I learn it?
- Why does it matter to me as a social worker?
- What will I do in my future social work practice, in light of this learning?

Critical thinking is expected throughout. You must establish relevance, accuracy, precision, and clarity in order to build depth, breadth, logic, significance and fairness. Lay and McGuire (2010) state that students have reported finding this model useful for challenging them to think critically and to develop their learning.

Adapted from Lay and McGuire 2010

3.6.3 Tool 3

The Toronto model (Bogo et al. 2011)

This is a useful tool when reflecting on an interview with service users. It was developed through research at the University of Toronto in Canada, to develop a mechanism to assess students' ability to demonstrate meaningful reflection. It is used there as a formal assessment tool but it can also be used formatively to self-monitor the development of reflection. There are three headings: use of self, conceptualisation of practice and learning and growth as a professional.

Use of self

1. How did you feel and what were you experiencing during the interview?
2. How did you use these feelings in the interview?
3. Can you think of any personal and/or professional experiences that influenced your approach to the interview?

Conceptualisation of practice

1. What were the main issues the service user was dealing with?
2. Can you think of something you have learnt?

3. Are there any ideas from other disciplines that influenced your approach during the interview?

4. Did issues related to diversity impact on your approach in the interview? Can you give an example?

5. If you continue to work with this service user, what theoretical approach(es) would you consider using?

6. Based on what you knew coming into the interview, was there anything unexpected in the interview? If so, what was your approach to dealing with this? How did you respond to this unexpected aspect of the interview?

7. What did you find most challenging about this case? What was your approach to dealing with this challenge?

Learning and growth as a professional

1. If you could do this interview again what would you do differently, if anything?

2. As you continue to see this service user, what would your next steps be?

3. What did you feel you learnt from this interview?

4. How might this learning experience influence your approach to other service users?

5. Do you have any final thoughts about the interview?

(Adapted from Bogo et al. 2011)

Bogo et al. (2011) have developed an assessment scale and this can be found in the published journal article as set out in *Further reading* at the end of this chapter.

 TOP TIP   Tips for activities or actions to support reflection

- Keep a reflective journal.
- Hold reflective conversation (this may help you to explore and debate issues which you had not previously considered).
- Examine your reaction to issues.
- Consider how others involved may describe the event.
- Analyse what influences may lead to the different perceptions of the event.
- Consider what you have learnt and what you need to develop further.

(Cooper et al. 2008)

3.7 BARRIERS TO REFLECTION

3.7.1 What are the possible barriers to reflection and how might you overcome them?

Students with whom we have worked and learnt alongside have told us that for some there are barriers to becoming a reflective practitioner. These include:

- Confusion about what the term reflection means.
- Uncertainty about *what* to reflect on.

- Lack of understanding about *how* to reflect.
- Finding the process of reflecting on your own thoughts, feelings and actions daunting, unsettling or upsetting because
  - it involves challenging beliefs and perspectives
  - it involves challenging information or workplace practices previously considered valid.
- Finding that the process of reflection leads to uncertainty or unknowing rather than greater clarity or understanding.

If you recognise any of the above, we can reassure you that most students feel the same at some point, and you may have to persevere to be able to be comfortable with reflection and reflective practice. Having someone to discuss reflection with is especially important – tutor, other students, colleagues or mentors. Reflection, if done well, *can* be unsettling, as it can lead us to challenge deep and personally held beliefs and assumptions as we begin to reframe our understanding by applying social work knowledge and values.

TOP TIP   Strategies for addressing these barriers

- Talk to other students about their understanding – often trying to explain a concept to someone else helps to sharpen your understanding and you may learn new ways of approaching the topic. Do remember, however, to clarify this with further reading, information provided by the programme team and by your practice educator.
- Arrange to talk to your lecturer/tutor/practice educator and engage in a conversation about gaining greater understanding of the principles and techniques involved or about the emotional impact of reflection.
- Practise by reflecting on a recent practice incident, or a university-based incident, using one of the tools set out above or the format provided on the course you are following.
- Try using different techniques – such as a mindmap, a blog or a reflective diary – until you find one that works best for you.
- Re-read the sections in this chapter that explain reflection; having thought about them or discussed them with other students or staff, this information may be clearer.

CONCLUSION

Reflection helps social workers to be flexible and responsive whilst drawing on their knowledge base, skills and social work values and using these in a way that is appropriate to the practice situation. Reflective skills enable a social worker to work effectively in areas that are complex, that cannot simply be solved by standardised administrative processes and that involves balancing power and discretion and use of self (Payne 2006).

The College of Social Work (2012 b) remind us that 'over time, social work practitioners should become highly skilled in this so that it is also possible to integrate the ability to critically analyse and reflect to the extent that one can apply the ability as you are making decisions. This is what people might call 'using professional judgement', and has in other places been termed 'reflection-in-action'.

We will conclude with the thoughts of a former social work student.

I have been thinking about how to explain reflection to current students. I have come up with the idea that reflection is the considering and 'unpacking' or deconstructing of an issue, an idea, an incident from a number of angles to understand it better and to move forward with a clearer understanding of how to practise in future. Sometimes reflection feels like a window onto my deeper feelings and beliefs that influence my interaction with others. It involves looking at some of the painful or uncomfortable feelings and thought processes that accompany regrets or mistakes but which helps me to move forward from them. It is a way of thinking about, processing and reframing things in order to develop or change beliefs and behaviour in order to be a better practitioner.

We wish you a productive and enlightening reflective journey.

FURTHER READING

Bogo, M., Regehr, C., Katz, E., Logie, C. and Mylopoulos, M. 2011. Developing a tool for assessing students' reflections on their practice. *Social Work Education* 30(2), 186–94.

Green Lister, P. and Crisp, B. 2007. Critical incident analyses: a practice learning tool for students and practitioners. *Practice* 19(1), 47–60.

Lay, K. and McGuire, L. 2010. Building a lens for critical reflection and reflexivity in social work education. *Social Work Education.* 29(5), 539–50.

CHAPTER 4
DEVELOPING CRITICAL THINKING AND CRITICAL WRITING SKILLS

This chapter will introduce you to the concepts of critical thinking and critical writing. By following the advice provided, and applying the techniques presented, you will be equipped to develop skills in critical thinking and critical analysis, of literature and situations.

IN THIS CHAPTER WE WILL:

1. Introduce you to the language of critical thinking and analysis.
2. Explain how to use a 'critical lens' to deepen your understanding.
3. Examine critical thinking and emphasise its importance in assignment writing and in social work practice.
4. Identify a range of techniques for developing critical thinking and critical writing.
5. Consider some of the techniques used by lecturers to support the development of critical thinking and critical writing.
6. Explain and provide examples of critical writing.

Critical thinking is important for all students on all social work programmes and it must be demonstrated in your university-based and practice-based work, in increasingly in-depth ways as you progress through the programme, in order to demonstrate 'graduateness'. On a postgraduate programme you are expected to apply these skills from the beginning.

Developing skills in critical thinking and critical writing will enable you to *demonstrate* your deepening knowledge and understanding of social work theories, concepts, values and ethics and practice in your assignments and achieve higher marks.

4.1 WHY IS IT IMPORTANT?

Critical thinking is the art of analysing and evaluating thinking with a view to improving it.

(Elder and Paul 2006)

Although service users, carers and employing organisations need social workers who are reflective practitioners (as we learnt about in Chapter 3), they also need social workers who can engage in critical thinking and writing. Critical thinking and critical writing are an integral part of the social work qualification as well as an essential skill when following a higher education programme of study.

In the introductory chapter you learnt about the Benchmarks for Social Work. It is set out in the Benchmarks for Social Work (QAA 2008 5.1) that honours graduates should

'acquire, critically evaluate, apply and integrate knowledge and understanding in the following five core areas of study.

- Social work services, service users and carers
- The service delivery context
- Values and ethics
- Social work theory
- The nature of social work practice.'

The Benchmarks contain several statements about critical thinking skills and other intellectual skills associated with this. Some of these skills are generic, that is they can be applied in any situation, and some are specifically about the practice of social work. The Benchmarks set out clearly what is expected of graduates of social work programmes. They should be able to

'**analyse and synthesise** knowledge gathered for problem-solving purposes, i.e. to:

- **assess human situations**, taking into account a variety of factors (including the views of participants, theoretical concepts, research evidence, legislation and organisational policies and procedures)
- **analyse information** gathered, weighing competing evidence and modifying their viewpoint in light of new information, then relate this information to a particular task, situation or problem
- **consider specific factors** relevant to social work practice (such as risk, rights, cultural differences and linguistic sensitivities, responsibilities to protect vulnerable individuals and legal obligations)
- **assess the merits** of contrasting theories, explanations, research, policies and procedures

- **synthesise knowledge and sustain reasoned argument**
- employ **a critical understanding** of human agency at the macro (societal), mezzo (organisational and community) and micro (inter- and intrapersonal) levels
- **critically analyse** and take account of the impact of inequality and discrimination in work with people in particular contexts and problem situations.

(QAA 2008: 5.5.3)

This may seem initially daunting but we can reassure you that these terms will become more familiar as you work through this chapter. However, it is not only important to acquire and demonstrate critical thinking and critical writing skills in order to pass the course and become a qualified social worker, but it is also essential in order to equip you with the personal and intellectual qualities to practise using a sensitive and ethical approach, based on a sound understanding of the complex and political nature of social work. This chapter will help you understand the terms used in the Benchmark statement and the Professional Capability Framework (PCF) and how to acquire and demonstrate these skills, and by doing so become a more effective learner *and* a more effective social worker.

It is set out in the PCF (College of Social Work 2012a) in the domain of *Critical Reflection and Analysis* that social workers:

are knowledgeable about and apply the principles of critical thinking and reasoned discernment. They identify, distinguish, evaluate and integrate multiple sources of knowledge and evidence. These include practice evidence, their own practice experience, service user and carer experience together with research-based, organisational, policy and legal knowledge. They use critical thinking augmented by creativity and curiosity.

At the end of the final placement a social work student should be able to:

- Apply imagination, creativity and curiosity to their practice.
- Inform decision-making through the identification and gathering of information from multiple sources, actively seeking new sources.
- With support, rigorously question and evaluate the reliability and validity of information from different sources.
- Demonstrate a capacity for logical, systematic, critical and reflective reasoning and apply the theories and techniques of reflective practice.
- Know how to formulate, test, evaluate and review hypotheses in response to information available at the time and apply in practice.

4.1.1 Is critical thinking the key to finding 'the right answer'?

Looking for 'the right answer' in assignments (other than if there is a multiple-choice test or exam as part of your assessment) will be a long, difficult and open-ended search. Reaching an awareness that there are lots of possible right or possible wrong answers depending on your standpoint and the evidence available is an important step in the process of learning to make informed judgements. In the contested area of social work knowledge, being able to weigh up the evidence to make judgements is an essential component of becoming a social worker. The starting point is curiosity, an enquiring mind and an ability to engage in problem solving. Critical thinking involves not just remembering and repeating what you have heard or read but re-processing the material. It is not simply about thinking and learning, but about adopting an approach that searches for and creates new meanings and new interpretations.

4.2 THE LANGUAGE OF CRITICAL THINKING AND CRITICAL ANALYSIS

You may not be surprised to learn that there is no agreed single definition of critical thinking. The work of Barnett (1997) on critical thinking fits well in a social work context. He recognises that there is both an intellectual and an emotional component to it, and that it is part of becoming a critical person in all aspects of life. This matches well with our view that critical thinking is not an isolated activity or set of techniques to be used when producing assignments; it is an integral part of being a critical social work practitioner. Your motivations for joining a social work programme will be varied, but are likely to involve a desire to 'make a difference' in some way. Through combining your personal qualities and your intellectual qualities you will find that developing a 'critical' approach becomes embedded in your professional identity, as you not only develop a critical viewpoint but also take action based on it.

You will come across the terms critical thinking, critical analysis, critical reasoning, critical awareness, critical practice as part of your social work qualification. As a student you may feel overwhelmed initially by these terms but we want to reassure you that they are all easily understood. They are all prefaced with *critical* – and the rest follows from there.

In everyday life the term 'critical' is used differently, often to mean negative criticism, whereas in an academic context it is taken to mean a critique of something, a consideration of and weighing up of all sides of an idea or situation in order to reach an informed and reasoned view. Sometimes students are initially wary of being critical and being asked to develop an argument, fearing that it is a one-sided approach or simply 'not done' to criticise authors of texts. In the academic sense, being critical is not about being 'negative' but about being sceptical, curious and open to new ideas and to reaching new understandings that are more detailed, informed and reasoned by weighing up arguments for and against and looking more closely at what is being said. By developing skills in critical thinking and critical analysis you are more likely not only to achieve higher marks, but also to develop a greater understanding of the realities of complex social work situations and be better equipped to intervene appropriately.

TOP TIP   Sarah's advice

When I first came across these terms with the word critical in them it was difficult to work out what they meant. Talking to my 'study buddy' helped. We also had large class discussions which reassured us that others felt the same and everyone's small contribution helped the group to understand the concepts and how to demonstrate them. Later I became excited by critical analysis – it helped me to understand and unpick complex situations. I gained confidence when I had positive feedback from the lecturers and my practice educator and after I saw that using critical thinking led to higher assignment marks. Now as a social worker I don't know how I would practise without having developed critical thinking skills. It certainly helps me understand complex situations more easily. It was worth persevering!

After you have worked through this chapter you may decide to refer to your 'study buddy' as your 'critical friend' instead.

4.3 LOOKING THROUGH A 'CRITICAL LENS'

As you have seen from the Benchmark statements and the PCF, social work involves working with complex situations, with no simple solutions, and in order to be effective as a practitioner it is important to view yourself, your practice, agency procedures, and the information about and provided by service users you are working with through what is often referred to as *a critical lens*. This does not mean being negative; it means that we should weigh up all the factors in order to reach a reasoned conclusion. Without this approach a social worker might resort to a single explanation for a problem and apply the same solution to a problem every time, whether it worked or not. Each person would receive similar services and there would be no consideration of the complex interaction between people and the wider societal influences on a person's life.

Case study:

Susie and Jon (1)

Susie is 19 years old, she is White British and lives alone in a two-bedroom flat in the town where she grew up and went to school. Susie has two children, neither of whom is living with her. Susie had a volatile relationship with the children's father; there was serious domestic violence and a chaotic lifestyle featuring substance use. Children's Services were involved with Susie during her childhood, and with both of her children. She is now in a relationship with Jon, aged 23, also of White British ethnicity. They are expecting their first child together. Jon has a son from a previous relationship whom he does not see. A referral was made to Children's Services by the Probation Service advising them of Susie's pregnancy. Jon is currently supervised by the Probation Service following a conviction of assault upon his ex-partner. Jon is known to Children's Services due to periods on a Child Protection Plan during his childhood, and latterly because of domestic violence with his ex-partner which compromised the safety of their child. Jon has a history of aggressive behaviour and social anxiety. He is a chronic cannabis user.

When you consider Sara and Jon's situation you may have noted how social work involves working with complex situations, with no simple solutions. In order to be effective as a practitioner it is important to view yourself, your practice, agency procedures, the information about service users from other professionals and the information from service users themselves through what we refer to as *a critical lens*. This means weighing up all the factors contributing to Susie and Jon's circumstances, looking beneath simple surface explanations and asking questions in order to reach a reasoned conclusion. We will be returning to the story of Susie and Jon later in the chapter.

You may believe that you don't yet know how to think or write critically. Following the guidance in this chapter will assist you to identify the skills you already have and to develop these skills further and to identify new approaches and techniques.

Take a moment to consider the definition of social work agreed by the International Federation of Social Workers (IFSW) and the International Association of Schools of Social Work (IASSW) (2004).

The social work profession promotes social change, problem solving in human relationships and the empowerment and liberation of people to enhance well-being. Utilising theories of human behaviour and social systems, social work intervenes at the point where people interact with their environments. Principles of human rights and social justice are fundamental to social work.

4.3.1 Let's try to look at this through a critical lens

At first glance this definition might seem very straightforward and inspiring. It highlights social change and problem solving, which may come as no surprise. However, when we look more closely, using our critical lens, we can begin to see that some of the terms used are 'contested' – that is they are not agreed on by everyone, they may have different interpretations and meanings, or be difficult to define and pin down. When we use a critical lens to look more closely things initially appear more complicated, fuzzy or blurred, but the critical lens then leads to clearer understanding and a sharper, more focussed, way of seeing.

So, by looking more closely we might begin to see that the definition appears very broad and can be interpreted as idealistic, and may or may not reflect your own experiences of social work, or even the media portrayal of what social work is or might be. For example, the terms empowerment and liberation are complex and not straightforward. You might begin to ask yourself what is 'empowerment' and what might 'liberation' involve? Is liberation something that you saw as a central part of your social work practice? Might this have a different value in different situations and perhaps in other parts of the world? Remember, this is an international definition and whilst social work is very diverse in the UK, it is much more so when we take international perspectives into account. The term 'well-being' initially might sound straightforward, but what exactly is it, who defines it – the social worker or the service user or carer, and how might we go about enhancing it? You may have heard the term 'human rights' being used, and accepted that all people have rights, but may not have stopped to consider what this might mean in social work practice when one person's rights may be achieved at the expense of those of another person.

We might also use our critical lens to ask what is missing from the definition. Social work practitioners might point to the constraints of limited resources. Receiving a service is dependent upon meeting the criteria for accessing services, and the funding to meet needs is often inadequately distributed and this may seem unjust.

When we begin to see through the fuzziness and initial blur, we see that there are many, often conflicting, forces at play. Social workers rarely intervene in situations where the answers are clear or where everyone is in agreement about potential solutions. People's lives are complex. People are multifaceted and their circumstances influenced by life experiences, relationships, oppression and discrimination, for example. Some people will embrace change, some will resist it, some have a greater capacity for resilience. This is what makes social work so challenging whilst being equally rewarding. Using a critical approach enables social workers to work between and within all these layers of a person's life or situation, to seek potential solutions to problems, difficulties and dilemmas, and to challenge structures and processes that create barriers.

Sometimes this fuzziness is described as 'knowing and unknowing', where you find yourself clear and certain about some aspects of a topic but at the same time unclear and uncertain, when things that seemed simple are revealed as being more complicated.

4.4 WHAT IS CRITICAL THINKING AND WHY IS IT IMPORTANT?

Thinking critically involves asking questions. It involves taking nothing at face value and always looking beyond the information presented, considering the arguments and counter-arguments. You may be familiar with and competent at multi-tasking and handling large quantities of material and information, and doing this through the use of information technology devices. An example of this might be using a search engine to search for information – a popular one is 'Google' – but not being able to judge which material is accurate, valid or reliable. As part of your programme of study you will be learning how to use databases, an aspect of the electronic university library facilities, to search for material in a more systematic way. Whilst this material has undergone some 'filtering' for authenticity reliability and validity, you will still need to apply critical thinking techniques to make judgements about the material you have identified. (We will return to the processes of analysing information in Chapter 5.) Critical thinking:

- closely considers the values, assumptions and beliefs that inform knowledge, theories, practice and research;
- questions and makes judgements about the relevance and validity of information;
- is the basis of good decision making;
- underpins ethical reasoning;
- is needed for practice in organisations if social workers are to retain their professional integrity in the face of pressure to become organisational apparatchiks;
- is fundamental to social work's defence against becoming agents of social control rather than agents of social change;
- is essential for effective, sensitive and anti-oppressive practice.

The pitfalls of taking information at face value, or literally, are highlighted by Brown and Rutter (2006) in the following example.

- John has an attention-deficit hyperactivity disorder.
- Hyperactivity decreases academic performance.
- Drug X reduces hyperactivity.
- Therefore if we prescribe drug X for John, his academic performance will improve.
- Try to practise applying a critical lens to the statement that John has an attention-deficit hyper-activity disorder.

You might ask what other factors might be involved, such as John's home situation, diet, additional learning needs, a lack of stimulation, how others respond to him. You might question the appropriateness or accuracy of a medical diagnosis and be concerned about the appropriateness of labelling children in this way and of prescribing drugs. You may wonder what research has been undertaken, what evidence there is for the drug being effective, and how theories of child development are being applied and what alternative approaches there might be.

This example demonstrates that assumptions based on a lack of critical thinking can lead to inappropriate conclusions and all too common errors in practical judgement. The assumption that a drug will help John at school fails to consider many other factors.

4.5 TECHNIQUES FOR CRITICAL THINKING

These are not necessarily new techniques as you may already use some of these to an extent when you read a broadsheet newspaper or listen to the news, when you listen to friends' accounts of their situation when they are seeking your advice, when we make choices between political parties, choices about healthy eating or how much alcohol is safe to consume. It is likely that you will already be using some aspects of critical thinking to make sense of and navigate through everyday situations. By building on these you will soon be able to think critically and achieve greater success in your university assignments.

TOP TIP   Techniques for critical thinking (1)

Critical thinking involves...

- Standing back from information
- Breaking things down into elements
- Examining in detail from many different angles
- Checking accuracy
- Looking for possible flaws in reasoning, evidence, or the way that conclusions are drawn
- Comparing the same issue from a different viewpoint
- Being able to see and explain why different people arrived at different conclusions
- Being able to argue why one set of opinions, results or conclusions is preferable to another
- Being on guard for devices (e.g. statistics) that encourage us to take questionsable statements at face value, or lure us into agreement.

In a generic guide to critical thinking skills Cottrell (2005: 2) describes critical thinking as a process and lists the features of critical thinking as follows:

- Identifying other people's positions, arguments and conclusions
- Evaluating the evidence for alternative points of view
- Weighing up opposing arguments and evidence fairly
- Being able to read between the lines
- Recognising techniques used to make certain positions more appealing
- Reflecting on issues in a structured way, bringing logic and insight to bear
- Drawing conclusions about whether the arguments are valid and justifiable, based on good evidence and sensible assumptions
- Presenting a point of view in a structured and clear, well-reasoned way that convinces others.

Try to use these features of critical thinking when preparing your next assignment. You will need to apply them to the reading you are undertaking and the notes you make from that reading, and use them to develop an assignment plan that demonstrates the critical thinking skills that you are developing.

4.5.1 Warning! Critical thinking has the power to change you and the people around you

Critical thinking is essentially about asking questions, considering the range of explanations and drawing well-considered conclusions. Doing this changes the way in which we view the world. It should lead to shifts in our own thinking, and change perceived norms within the groups of people we associate with – our families and our friends. This can provoke anxiety in others as it challenges long-held beliefs or family traditions. As you develop and apply your critical lens you will find that assumptions, beliefs, values and social structures are all questioned, regardless of their originally perceived status, authority or assumed accuracy. Applying this to your own practice or ideas can be uncomfortable. It may result in a realisation that you had previously held what you recognise to be oppressive views or the recognition that you have reinforced inaccurate or negative social structures and attitudes. These changes in your perceptions and beliefs can lead to feelings of uncertainty. Learning to work with uncertainty and ambiguity can be uncomfortable and confusing. We advise that you seek support from your personal tutor/academic advisor if you are distressed about any views that you may be challenging and changing.

STUDENT EXPERIENCES

Often when students first join the social work programme, they consider themselves not to have prejudices or act or think in a discriminatory way. Through group discussions, class lectures and reading the course texts they find that their long-held views are being challenged which can lead to feeling unsettled and confused. This includes their understandings about the role of men and women, about race and religion, about family structures, about the newspapers they and their family and friends read and the links between newspapers and political parties. This leads to some interesting and awkward conversations with friends and family as they test out their new understanding. During practice placements they recognise that their views and assumptions continue to be challenged and new ways of viewing situations and people develop. When they feel uncomfortable they share their feelings with the friends they have made at university, and with their academic advisor/personal tutor. As newly qualified social work practitioners they continue to use and develop critical thinking skills, their critical lens, as an integral part of their day-to-day practice. It becomes embedded in the way they think and make decisions.

The ability to think critically is arguably the most important skill a social worker can possess and it is essential that you develop this skill as early as possible within your social work training. Having said this, the ability to write critically can take time to develop, and many students find this a difficult skill to learn and demonstrate in their writing. Good critical writing generally contributes to achieving higher marks.

Example

Sarah and Matt were puzzled at first about the range of new academic and professional skills they were expected to develop. They realised that they already possessed some aspects of critical thinking skills but hadn't thought of them in these terms. They also recognised that they were using some of the techniques of critical thinking without being conscious of it. In class discussions they recognised themselves as being curious about the world, sceptical of accepting information at face value and were open to looking at issues from different viewpoints and finding new and creative solutions to problems.

4.6 HOW DO THE TEACHING AND LEARNING STRATEGIES EXPERIENCED AT UNIVERSITY HELP TO DEVELOP CRITICAL THINKING?

4.6.1 The role of questions in teaching and learning

To develop critical thinking you need to adopt a questionsing attitude and approach to the ideas and scenarios that you are working with. In the university-based aspects of the programme, you will experience being asked questions by the teaching staff to help to develop a critical approach.

Remember, with the emphasis on active learning, you will be expected to participate in class and to have read key texts, chapters, papers etc. in preparation. The lecturer will ask questions, not because they have not prepared enough material to fill the time, but because they are rehearsing with you the steps for critical thinking and critical analysis and encouraging active and deeper learning.

During the practice-based aspects of the programme you will also be encouraged to demonstrate critical thinking and you will be expected to engage in structured discussions with your practice educator, to ask questions and to use a critical lens when learning about the agency, the team and the work undertaken with service users and carers.

Moon (2005: 16) sums this up well when she says that the classroom or seminar room should be 'a place where risk-taking is tolerated. It is a place for the exploration of ideas, rather than the simple transmission of knowledge, it is a place in which there is time to tease out problems rather than jump to a solution'.

So how might this happen?

Example

Here are some techniques that might be used by the lecturer in class to support the development of critical thinking.

The lecturer has delivered a short lecture with multimedia resources on this week's topic in the unit she is teaching to first year students. The lecturer takes a research-minded approach to her teaching and wants to make her lectures lively and engaging and to create a learning environment that supports learning and understanding. Using techniques from a model that she has read recently by Golding (2011) the lecturer asks questions during a teaching session such as:

- Why might that be? What explanations or reasons are offered by the authors you have read? (Students are invited to give reasons)

When students offer possible explanations, based on their reading, the lecturer might ask more questions to draw out more learning, for example:

- Can you explain in more detail what you mean? Can you give an example from your reading or from your practice? (Students are invited to clarify and explain)

Marija and Pavinder are students in this class and have each given an example from the reading or from their practice experience; the lecturer then might then ask:

- What are the differences and similarities between the ideas that Marija and Pavinder have offered?

Opening up the class discussion further she might then ask:

- What are the different perspectives offered in the reading that you have undertaken? Which arguments put forward in the literature are strongest/weakest and why? (Students are invited to compare)

This style of questioning helps to arrive at a clearer understanding of the material that has been covered in class. The questions do not simply ask students to repeat what they have read but to begin to critique the material.

Here are some examples of the types of questions you might be asked by the lecturer in order to develop a range of critical thinking skills when formulating your responses. You might not be asked to respond to the lecturer directly but to discuss these questions in pairs or small groups, and the lecturer may move around the room talking to groups and encouraging thought processes. Sharing different points of view can help to gain a clearer understanding of the possibilities of the topic you are learning about. Weighing up the alternative views can help you to look differently at the material and develop new insights as you begin to see that there appears to be no 'right' answer and that lots of answers are possible in different circumstances. You may then be asked to share some answers with the whole class and a further debating of the responses may take place.

These types of questions might also be asked by your practice educator when meeting to discuss the work you are engaged in during your practice learning placement.

Initiating	What questions might we ask about this topic or situation?
Suggesting	What are some possible ideas about this topic or situation? What are other alternatives?
Reasoning and elaborating	If ... were true what would follow from that ...? How might we explain more about ...? What is a different way of saying ...? What do you mean by ...? What is an example of ...?
Evaluating	Why do you think ...? What evidence is there for ...? What do you agree with and why? What do you disagree with and why? What is an alternative perspective?
Concluding	What conclusions can you draw? What needs to be done next?

(Adapted from Golding 2011: 362)

You will have seen that responding to the lecturer's or practice educator's questions involves being prepared for the class or meeting by having read the recommended reading for that session or the relevant placement documents, listening carefully and making a written or mental note of the things you are unclear about or want to clarify or explore further. This is sometimes described as taking responsibility for your own learning, and not expecting the lecturer or practice educator to simply tell you what you need to know in order to pass the assessment for that unit of study.

Some students arrive at university expecting to be given a lot of information by experts in their field and to be able to sit back, listen and memorise the information. It is important to participate in class, to share your experience and insights, to ask questions that help you to reinforce your understanding and at the same time helping others to clarify their thinking. Questions can also be asked when you are curious to find out more about a topic, as well as to clarify a point that you were not clear about. You will discover that a dynamic learning environment is created by doing this, and that knowledge is not a static thing but something that is jointly evolved and constructed by everyone in the class.

Being an active learner involves being proactive and a commitment to be an increasingly independent learner. This involves learning how to use the university library resources, both physical and online, setting aside time to read key and recommended texts, participating in class, and managing your time effectively. This will give you a firm foundation for developing critical thinking skills.

Useful skills for critical thinking:

- inquiring;
- problem solving;
- argument analysis and construction;

- uncovering and evaluating assumptions;
- justification;
- interpretation; and
- questioning

(Golding 2011: 360)

Stop and think time

Another strategy sometimes used by lecturers is to have a break in the timetabled session for students to pause and make quick notes summarising the key points and noting down areas for clarification. This then might be shared in pairs or small groups. It might be followed by an 'any questions' activity, possibly with the answers typed into a live document and archived on the virtual learning environment for future reference, or used to identify the literature search and additional reading that needs to be carried out by students before the next session. The lecturer may focus on generating questions rather than providing answers, as a step towards critical thinking.

Debates

Some lecturers use pre-planned class debates in which everyone participates in order to engage students in drawing out the arguments 'for and against'. The evidence is then summarised and conclusions drawn – following some of the steps of critical thinking.

Seminars

Seminars where set reading is required in advance are common, as a strategy for discussion in a smaller group than the whole class sessions. The lecturer may have asked you to read particular chapters of a book or books and papers from peer-reviewed journals, and to listen to or watch a service user's account of their experience of a situation. There may be some pre-set questions as triggers for the seminar, and you may have attended a lecture on that topic. You will be expected to prepare by making notes and to contribute to the discussion by sharing your insights rather than repeating what you have heard or read.

Looking for the 'right answer' will be a long, difficult and open-ended search. Reaching an awareness that there are lots of possible right or possible wrong answers depending on your standpoint and the evidence available is an important step in the process of learning to make informed judgements. In the contested area of social work knowledge, being able to weigh up the evidence to make judgements is an essential component of becoming a social worker. The starting point is curiosity, an enquiring mind and an ability to engage in problem solving. (Chapter 5 provides some technique and tools for analysing information.)

4.6.2 But how do I use my critical lens and question the work of famous people and published authors?

You may initially be puzzled about how to go about questioning the work of published authors and well-known thinkers. You may not feel confident to be able to do this, and may believe that what they have said is 'right' and indisputable. But as you will have discovered from your learning on the social work programme different authors hold views that appear to contradict or challenge the views of others, and offer differing theories about the same topic. You may ask yourself whether this means none of them are right, or whether they are only partly right, or if each approach helps to shed light on a problem or situation from a different angle. For example, you may be learning about the classic work of Freud. It is important to be aware that his ideas were developed in a previous century, using middle class white Europeans as subjects, and it is important to consider this when looking at the applicability of his ideas to contemporary social work. On the other hand, some published work may be 'out of date' in terms of the context whilst the underpinning ideas may still be relevant. This can initially feel complex and confusing.

Example

In Anne's experience as a social work lecturer, how to question and comment on the work of authors in the textbooks they are reading, particularly when there are conflicting viewpoints in the literature, is something students are concerned about. She offers reassurance by advising and encouraging them to approach it by using the following phrases as triggers and ways of organising the apparently conflicting material.

Phrases to use include:

- In this situation the evidence for ... is stronger/weaker/more compelling than the evidence for ... for the following reasons
- On the other hand ...
- The evidence provided by ... does not take into account ...
- On balance ...

These techniques are a good starting point from which to gain confidence in critiquing the work of 'famous people'.

4.6.3 Let's practice looking at some more material through a critical lens

A report by the National Institute for Clinical excellence (NICE 2004) indicated that depression is more common in women than men. It states that 1 in 4 women will suffer depression compared to 1 in 10 men and that social work resources directly aimed at the mental health of women are needed. A gendered approach with the main aim of tackling the morbidity rates amongst this over-represented gender group is proposed.

Let's consider how we might engage in critical thinking about this passage.

List the questions you might ask as a result of applying a critical lens and using critical thinking skills.

The following questions could be asked. Are they similar to the ones you have listed?

1. Does the above statement demonstrate clear and undisputed facts or are there areas which could be further discussed and examined?

2. How were the statistics gathered?

3. Are there other factors at play? For example, is it possible that women go to their GP more readily than men do to discuss feelings of depression?

4. Do men choose not to acknowledge they are experiencing feelings of depression?

5. Do GPs respond differently to men and women with the same symptoms?

6. How does gender affect mental health? Are women really more likely than men to experience depression? How might I find out more?

7. How accurate are the findings? Is everyone experiencing depression diagnosed?

8. What other explanations might there be? For example, what about other research which highlights alcohol as a possible form of self-medication for men?

9. Is this the whole story? Are the higher suicide rates amongst men an indicator that depression is more prominent than these figures suggest?

10. Consider the information from a particular viewpoint, for example a feminist position. Feminists may argue that this is evidence of women's oppression or that different language or labels are used when referring to the same symptoms in men in order not to label them as weak. Is there an assumption that women require professional support whereas men will cope alone?

11. Are there alternative statistics which may challenge or support the conclusion?

12. Do men and women subconsciously conform to certain gender roles applied by society? Does this influence their understanding of their own mental health?

13. Are people with depression receiving an appropriate and accurate diagnosis?

14. Are we being persuaded here to assume that men are the stronger sex and so do not experience depression?

15. Do the findings justify the recommendations? Might there be other recommendations from the same findings?

16. Do the conclusions consider other factors which may influence these findings, such as different helping-seeking behaviour amongst men?

Some of these critical questions can be asked by simply reading the information we provided. Some of the questions could only be asked by searching for and reading additional material about depression.

Without this fuller understanding of the competing themes and issues that wider reading and critical thinking brings, decisions will be based on a possible combination of incomplete or inaccurate information, second-hand knowledge and stereotypes. It is essential that you spend time reading around your subject, looking for competing theories and additional research studies. Achieving a broader and more critical view of the literature available will enable you to demonstrate the acquisition and application of critical thinking in assignments and will contribute to higher marks as long as you have also paid attention to the assignment guidelines and the learning outcomes for this piece of work. Always check the general information about assignments provided in the programme handbook, the written guidance for that particular assignment and any supplementary advice from the lecturer or practice educator.

TOP TIP   Techniques for critical thinking (2)

- Take nothing at face value.
- Acknowledge the impact of your beliefs and ideologies – challenge their accuracy.
- Acknowledge the meaning behind your feelings.
- Identify examples to illustrate your arguments.

- Provide evidence from wider reading for your arguments.
- Try to break down complex ideas into their component parts.
- Seek out alternative points of view.
- Identify and weigh up the arguments used to support the opposing perspectives.
- Be aware of your blind spots or prejudices – and how they might be influencing your critique.

By this stage you should have a better understanding of what critical thinking is and its importance to social work. In order to achieve success in the social work programme you need to be able to apply critical thinking in a variety of situations and assignment formats. During the early stages of the undergraduate degree you will not be expected to write with highly developed critical skills. However, this is not to say that you should not develop these skills as early as possible. We will now explore what critical writing looks like.

4.7 WRITING CRITICALLY

Typical feedback on student assignments from the markers will often include statements such as 'more analysis of the themes needed' or 'it is important to include critique rather than description'. But what does this actually mean and how can students develop this essential skill?

The starting point for writing critically is being able to think critically. Critical thinking underpins critical writing. Both skills go hand in hand; neither operates without the other. However, some people are better able to express their thoughts in writing. If you find you are having difficulty expressing your ideas after you have read study skills books like this one, we strongly recommend that you find out about study skills workshops available to you at the university where you are studying. Setting your ideas down on paper – or on the screen – provides an opportunity to further critique your ideas as you read and re-read what you have produced. We still refer to this as writing, even though you are more likely to be typing! Some assessments involve collaborative group work and a group assignment and you may have an opportunity to comment on drafts before submitting the completed assignment. This provides a valuable opportunity to apply more than one critical lens to the work. You might feel daunted initially about sharing your work with other people in your class, but it is important to remember that other students will also have similar feelings and to be constructive in your comments to them. It might help to remember that in social work practice your writing is not 'private' or 'hidden' as you will be completing assessments, reports, case recording and sharing them with colleagues and it is useful practice to develop a clear 'written' style.

When you first write an assignment you may find you are using a descriptive style, setting out what you have read but not being able to judge the relative importance of the material in order to reach your own conclusions, particularly when the authors you have read may offer differing approaches to the same problem, situation or topic. For example, you may have read about several different schools of thought in psychology and sociology, a range of social work interventions such as crisis intervention, task-centred practice and group work. You may have found it difficult at first to distinguish between them and then feel confident enough to be able to describe them in your own words. You then may have used your critical lens and the checklists and tips we have shared with you to interpret them when applied to a range of different situations or scenarios. Using critical thinking processes helps you to develop and present an argument based on weighing up the information and choosing a particular course of action or a particular conclusion in a given situation, and your arguments might be informed by particular ideology, for example a feminist or Marxist analysis that offers a view of the world that you personally identify with.

Example

Here we use the scenario of a conversation between you and a friend about a film you have seen to illustrate the difference between description and critical analysis. You might explain the film by **describing** the plot from beginning to end, picking out some key scenes and explaining what each character said and what happened. You might describe the location or the humour, or how good-looking the actors were.

On the other hand you might explain to your friend why you preferred this particular film over another. You might give a brief synopsis of the main plot, and the style (or genre), the director and why those actors suited the part, and any unusual techniques used, and why the film was constructed in this way. By approaching it this way you are applying critical thinking skills, by **analysing** the significance of some aspects of the film and relating this to other areas of your film knowledge. By taking a *critical* stance, very much how film critics approach their work, you are likely to begin to compare the films and explain why one film was 'better' than the other. The conversation might end with a recommendation of which one your friend should see and the reasons why.

Let's apply this to academic writing. You need to set the scene for the conversation – the introduction. This would be fairly short. Some defining of the terms may be helpful but this is not always necessary as you can assume that the lecturer, as with an experienced film-goer, will understand the key terms used. The main body will consist of analysis of the themes, not a descriptive blow-by-blow account of who said what and where and what happened next. As in a conversation about films, some description to set the context or illustrate a pivotal moment, underlying theme or motive can be useful. The conclusion might recommend a particular film over another, or recommend an alternative that combines aspects of other films or a film that represents a new genre or interpretation. It is important to include an accurate reference list – in the case of a film you would want enough information to be able to identify the films referred to in order to watch them yourself.

Often students struggle to keep the descriptive writing to a minimum, particularly in the beginning when learning how to write effective assignments. They will often use valuable word allocations to describe a topic. This may be for two reasons. Firstly, there are many introductory texts written in an accessible style that explain social work topics rather than critiquing them. The texts that critique the material may be seen by students to be complex and difficult to understand until they have become more familiar with the topic. This involves spending a lot of time reading around the subject in order to develop an understanding of the topic. Secondly, students often believe that by describing something they are demonstrating to the lecturers marking the assignment that they have read it and understood it. Using description demonstrates you can reproduce what you have read, but does not demonstrate whether you have understood the literature and the themes and debates contained within it – it does not demonstrate your problem-solving skills that are so important in social work practice.

You may want to watch a film critic on TV to see how concisely they evaluate the films and then consider how you could apply critical analysis to the assignments you are preparing.

Case study:

Susie and Jon (2)

Here we see how a student has attempted to critically analyse some of the issues in relation to the case study about Susie and Jon rather than simply describing them.

> Significantly Brofenbrenner (1989) added an additional aspect to the model, the chrono-system which recognised the importance of placing historical context as it occurs in the different systems. For example, the history of Susie and Jon's own parent–child relationships is likely to influence the current situation but may not be obviously evident from their existing dynamics.

> Although Brofebrenner's principles promote a rounded model of assessment, Swick and Williams (2006: 371) advise we must use his construct with his own caution of 'do no harm' to families. They see the model as an opportunity to build empowering relationships within families, and to use the model effectively we must avoid 'categorising, stereotyping, and impeding families through the work and relations we develop with them' (Swick and Williams 2006: 371). These principles are a cornerstone of social work practice and my personal values; nevertheless, I am mindful that whilst it is necessary for me to build a relationship with Susie and Jon and listen to their story, it is impera- tive that I remain focussed on safeguarding their baby. An Ofsted report evaluating serious case reviews (SCRs) revealed that in some of the SCRs, the safeguarding implications for the child had been overlooked because too much attention had been focussed on the parents; especially when they were themselves vulnerable (Ofsted 2011).

Lecturer comment

It is clear that the writer is approaching this with an understanding of the deeper issues involved, drawing on wider literature to justify the points being made. Critical thinking is demonstrated, with an acknowledgement of social work values.

4.7.1 Descriptive and critical writing

Here we have provided some short examples to illustrate the differences between descriptive and critical writing.

Descriptive writing	Critical writing
Describes something:	Critiques something:
The Fairer Access to Care Services policy (FACS) provides local authorities with guidance on the principles to follow regarding access to care for adults. Its aim is to ensure a more consistent eligibility decision across the country. It encourages local authorities to set a low threshold when deciding whose needs should be met. It takes a proactive approach to widening access to care for adults.	The Fairer Access to Care Services (FACS) policy provides local authorities with guid- ance on the principles to follow regarding access to care for adults. It aims to ensure a consistent eligibility decision across the country. However, as local authorities can set their own threshold there is a risk that there will be different outcomes for assessed need depending on where some- one lives, leading to what is often referred to as a 'post code lottery' and negating the aim to ensure consistency.

Descriptive writing	Critical writing
Explains something:	Explains its relevance to social work:
Maslow's Hierarchy of Needs sets out several levels of need in a triangular model. People must begin with basic needs such as the physiological need for food, clothes and shelter. Maslow suggests that to achieve what he describes as self-actualisation (fulfilling potential), the apex of the triangle, a person must first meet lower needs.	Theories such as Maslow's Hierarchy of Needs can inform social work assessments. Maslow sets out seven stages of need, which he suggests people must navigate through in sequential order, starting with a need for food, clothes and shelter, before they can fulfil their potential. There are limitations to this theory. For example, it is possible that some people would sacrifice food or shelter for the pursuit of creativity. However, such theories offer an optional framework, rather than a strict template, by which to consider human need. Considering individual differences and preferences, rather than strictly applying this hierarchical model will enable social workers to consider where resources may be best used to achieve change.

The extracts below, from student assignments, demonstrate differences in writing descriptively and critically.

Important: These are intended as illustrations of the differences between the two styles of writing rather than as model answers. You must *not* copy them in to assignments that you are preparing. Remember, there are strict rules about plagiarism and your university handbook will contain information about this and it is essential that you follow these rules.

Example 1

(a) Descriptive writing

The social model explains mental illness in terms of the impact a person's social class, social support, isolation and poverty has on their mental wellbeing. This theory states that any positive or negative change to a person's life can affect their psychological wellbeing (Gibb and Macpherson 2000). The Black Report (1980) highlighted the effect of social class on medical morbidity; stating that unskilled people of low social class were at twice as much risk of death than someone of higher social class. The social model of mental illness links isolation to psychiatric disorders such as schizophrenia and depression, and to stress and suicidal behaviour. Thompson (2000) suggests that the social model of health is more closely aligned to social work values; it should therefore be used in social work practice.

(b) Critical writing

Practitioners worldwide cannot agree on why mental illness occurs. Social constructionists argue that mental disorder is socially constructed and challenge whether it actually exists (Busfield 2001). They argue that the very notion of mental disorder is constructed by the psychiatric profession as a way of medicating and so controlling deviant behaviour. Brown (1995) aims criticism at social constructionism as a theory, suggesting it is limited by refusing to accept any elements of structural perspectives, in particular the notion that fundamental social structures of society play key roles in health and illness. Social causation theories, unlike social construction, essentially accept constructs such as schizophrenia and depression as a legitimate diagnosis. However, the emphasis within this approach is upon the relationship between social disadvantage and mental illness (McPherson 2000). Brown (1995) argues that to begin to understand mental illness, both explanations are needed, arguing that both ideologies allow individuals to look beyond the surface level of any one problem. Both theories are significant to social work as together they enable professionals to gain a better understanding of why people experience mental ill health. As eluded to by Rogers and Pilgrim (2005), no one explanation has ever been agreed; this therefore gives credence to a pluralist understanding, influenced by both models.

Example 2

(a) Descriptive writing

The National Institute for Clinical Excellence (2004) states that 1 in 4 women will suffer from depression compared with 1 in 10 men. There is evidence that more women are treated for mental health problems than men (National Statistics 2003). Symptoms normally display themselves in the same way whether a person is male or female. The most common symptoms are poor mood, lethargy, poor appetite, lack of enthusiasm and a poor sleep pattern.

(b) Critical writing

It is problematic to accurately measure whether men or women experience higher rates of depression. Figures from the National Institute for Clinical Excellence (2004) and from National Statistics (2003) indicate that more women than men required treatment for a mental ill-health condition, with 1 in 4 women compared to 1 in 10 men being diagnosed with depression. However, this research only measured known diagnosed cases. It is possible that men find other ways of coping without professional help, and remain unaccounted for in these statistics as other sources (National Statistics 2001) indicated that 80% of people dependent upon alcohol were male. This may indicate that men use alcohol as a form of self-medication (Volkow 2004). Furthermore, Moller-Leimkuhler (2003) inform us that the male suicide rate is twice as high in the UK and six times more likely in the US compared to suicide rates for women. Arguably social workers need to remain open to the possibility that a large proportion of male depression remains undiagnosed and untreated, that alcohol misuse might mask depression, and that depression might be a factor in male suicide.

As you can see, writing critically involves moving beyond description. You will begin to gain confidence in your ability to think and write critically as you gain more practice in assignment writing, and in particular in:

- knowing your subject, and becoming familiar with the arguments and counter-arguments;
- using a *sociological imagination* and viewing the world through a critical lens;
- looking at the same issue from the perspective of different theories and writers;
- exploring the evidence for different conclusions;
- considering the implications, and in particular the practice implications, of the conclusions drawn.

Case study:

Susie and Jon (3)

Here is an extract from an assignment that considered the case study involving Susie and Jon. Identify the aspects which demonstrate critical thinking and critical writing, using one of the numbered techniques for critical thinking that are included in this chapter.

> In the wake of concerns that follow a serious case review such as Baby P (LSCB Haringey 2009), there is an understandable increase in public and professional anxiety, broad critical reflection, and often changes in systems, structures and practice aimed at trying to prevent a repeat event. For example, since the death of Baby P (Peter Connelly) in 2007 there has been more than a 50% rise in applications to court to remove children from their parents, referred to as the 'Baby Peter effect' (Hall & Guy 2009). The NSPCC has commented that the rise was likely to be because people were now 'more alert to situations where children are at risk' (Adams 2012). In addition to this, I would argue that latterly the increase reflects the effect of financial cuts to support services designed to keep children safe within their own family, together with a move towards more risk adverse defensive social work practice. A move, perhaps driven by local authority management to avoid public criticism and social worker's fear of individual blame when a case goes 'wrong'. Certainly in my work place I often hear the comment 'I don't want to be the one ending up in court over this'.

This is an example of how the wider cultural influences of the media, placed within the exo-system of society, directly affects social work practice. It explains in part why 'risk' has become a dominant preoccupation within the Western society in the latter part of the 20th century, to the point where Beck (1992) describes us living in a 'risk society' with an emphasis on uncertainty, individualisation and culpability. As a result, risk assessment has become embedded within the assessment process and is associated with negativity despite risk being a normal and beneficial part of everyday life. However, whilst it of course enables a child's learning and development, in the context of child protection, some risks may need to be monitored, and at times restricted. The debate therefore is how best to assess risk, and moreover how to manage it in the least oppressive way.

Jon's childhood chronology informs us that his early experiences were beleaguered by domestic violence and instability due to frequent moves to escape abuse, but then returning to the same situation. The impact of Jon's childhood on his behaviour towards Susie, and his parenting style, needs to be explored. Bentovim et al. (2009, p.183) state that

> 'the degree of stability and protection the parents had as children in their own development, and the range of adverse experiences they suffered including exposure to violence and abuse and loss and the way they relate to past experiences can affect their current functioning'.

Whilst it is important for me to consider, with Jon, what his childhood script means for him and how this influences his patterns of behaviour, I am mindful not to assume it fully explains his violence towards women, or indeed to excuse it. It would be simplistic to apply the explanation of cyclical behaviour to all children exposed to trauma. Indeed Humphreys (2006, p.3) makes the point that practitioners should be wary of the 'notions of cycles of abuse which predict that children living with domestic violence will grow up to be violent'.

Humphreys (2006, p.3), notes that research has identified very individual reactions from children who live with domestic violence, and therefore we must not to assume permanent psychological damage has occurred Some children appear to thrive despite their negative circumstances and evolve various strategies to overcome adversity. This is often referred to as a person's resilience and is an integral part of our individuality.

4.7.2 Monitoring your progress

You can monitor your progress and critique your own assignments using the checklist below before you submit your work. Take advantage of opportunities to receive additional feedback on how to improve your assignment writing, for example discussing your mark and feedback with the lecturer who marked the work to pick up additional tips and advice on how to increase your marks in future assignments.

TOP TIP   Techniques for critical thinking (3)

Checklist of activities associated with critical thinking in academic writing	Does my assignment contain this?
Providing in-depth explanation (not description) of a subject or practice issue including considering strengths and weaknesses	A lot/a little/not at all
Exploring explanatory frameworks (theory and models) along-side other areas of evidence (research, statistics, professional experience), make judgements about the strength, validity and accuracy for the subject area	A lot/a little/not at all
Provide new ideas based on independent thinking or practice experience and values – assess their validity in comparison to the major perspectives on the subject	A lot/a little/not at all
Transfer practice/knowledge/theory from other situations to provide alternative solutions to the current issue. Consider the impact of 'doing nothing', the so what of critical thinking	A lot/a little/not at all
Explore outcomes and make judgements based on evidence. Draw together the thinking to provide a summary of the critical appraisal	A lot/a little/not at all

(Adapted from Brown and Rutter 2006: 14)

We recognise that writing critically is daunting for students. However, Moon (1999) considers the purpose of writing in terms of learning to think and reflect critically as an activity in itself. This is because writing involves the framing and reframing of a particular issue or idea. The process compels students to take time to think, and rethink from a number of different angles. It can engage our deeper learning by slowing down our thought processes as we attempt to put our ideas on paper and ensure our understanding by our attempt to explain the concept or conflict accurately. By slowing down our thinking, writing (or typing) enables us to consider other connections or new ideas as we find ourselves engaging in critical thinking.

Using a critical perspective within assignments becomes more important as you move through the programme.

Let's explore what you might wish to accomplish at each stage.

Sarah's targets for undergraduate year one included:

- 'Exploring major social work perspectives, reading around the subjects and formulating my own viewpoints.
- Preparedness and willingness to engage in critical thinking.
- Questioning previously held beliefs.

- Reading, listening to and considering a range of viewpoints and their relative merit.
- Gaining confidence in reflecting with others and discussing my views and arguments – finding my 'voice'.
- Developing an interest in current affairs – and applying my new learning to deconstruct arguments and information.
- Considering the importance of critical thinking in relation to ethics and values in social work.'

By aspiring to become curious and more open-minded Elder and Paul (2006) consider students at this phase to be moving from an unawareness of issues in their thinking towards becoming a *'challenged thinker'*, that is, one who is conscious of the flawed thinking they may experience.

Matt's targets for undergraduate year two included:

- 'Beginning to link critical thinking with practice interventions and develop an awareness of critical practice.
- Awareness of the range of options rather than simply attempting to find one answer or solution.
- Being able to critique literature and situations by applying a range of techniques.
- Beginning to consider my own practice through engaging in critical thinking, critical writing and reflection.
- Understanding the value of creativity in social care planning and problem solving alongside routine tasks.
- Developing an understanding of the personal, organisational and societal influences on social work practice.
- Reducing my reliance on the search for concrete answers.'

During this level of the programme students will normally develop a heightened awareness of the importance of critical thinking. They will be expected to be thinking critically in lectures, assignments and in practice during their placement. Students will normally be beginning to *practise* critical thinking on a regular basis and will be doing this through engaging in debate and discussion with the lecturers, peers and placement staff. Feedback on assignments should be thoughtfully considered and recommendations acted upon. Discussing the feedback with the marker, where this is possible, may help you to consider how to further develop and demonstrate your critical thinking and writing skills.

A social work lecturer normally expects to see the following being demonstrated at undergraduate final year:

- Routinely linking critical thinking with practice interventions through a developed awareness of critical practice.
- Becoming proficient at understanding contradictory evidence with an awareness of the range of options rather than simply attempting to find one answer or solution.
- Being able to critique literature and situations by applying a range of techniques with confidence.
- Actively and regularly considering your own practice through engaging in critical thinking, critical writing and reflection.
- Engaging in, where appropriate, creativity in problem solving alongside routine tasks.
- Demonstrating a detailed understanding of the personal, organisational and societal influences on social work practice.
- Having an open-minded and alternative approach to problem solving.
- Paying attention to feelings and reflecting on their meaning and influence on social work practice.

In addition, the following academic skills are expected to be demonstrated at master's level:

- In-depth knowledge of the subject area using current research and ideas with evidence of extensive independent study and independent thinking.
- Able to recognise, reconcile and work with complexity and contradictions.
- Demonstrate critical judgement, synthesis of information and ideas and the development of new ideas and solutions.
- Rigorous structured arguments communicated effectively.

Final year undergraduate and master's-level students are becoming independent learners, using independent thinking in preparation for practice as a newly qualified social worker. Thinking has become more advanced. Critical reflection has developed to become 'second nature' through questioning of self and the world. This will stand you in good stead as newly qualified social workers ready to engage in practice situations that are often characterised by uncertainty, complexity, risk and constant change.

TOP TIP

You may wish to construct your own checklist, based on the assessment criteria provided by the institution you are studying at for the level of the programme appropriate to you.

TOP TIP   Techniques for critical thinking (4)

A social work lecturer (Heron 2006) undertook some research into how social work students on four programmes in Scotland demonstrated critical thinking and critical writing in their assignments in the early stages of their programme. The framework used to consider whether the assignments contained critical writing that demonstrated critical thinking was as follows:

1. unpacking concepts – ability to break down ideas, concepts or theories;
2. recognising contradictions – differentiating between viewpoints and counter-arguments;
3. development – explaining a phenomenon, joining ideas together to form lines of arguments;
4. providing evidence – supporting or justifying assertions;
5. examining implications of evidence – generating hypotheses about consequences or examining the relationships between key factors;
6. alternative interpretation – questionsing or challenging an interpretation of the evidence and offering an alternative.

This is a further useful tool to demonstrate critical writing in your own assignments underpinned by critical thinking.

CONCLUSION

Critical thinking involves extending your knowledge and learning in order to transfer understanding from one situation to another whilst promoting social work values. It is helpful to reflect on the assignments you have produced and the social work interventions you have been involved in, in order to improve future assignments and interventions. Social workers use critical thinking skills to identify and counter assumptions or prejudices to ensure their own belief systems and previous life experiences do not colour their viewpoint, or assessments, of the individuals, groups or families they work with. By gaining experience and confidence in critical thinking, students and practitioners can avoid becoming complacent 'it has always been done this way' or defensive 'it worked last time' in their practice. Using critical thinking to underpin practice will help develop innovative, creative practitioners who are able to reframe circumstances in order to consider alternative perspectives and solutions. Importantly, students who adopt a critical approach to their studies and practice will combine this with critical reflection (see Chapter 3) in order to develop professional, accountable and effective social work services for service users and carers.

FURTHER READING

Fook, J. 2012. *Social work; a critical approach to practice*. 2nd ed. London: Sage.

Jones, S. 2009. *Critical learning for social work students*. London: Sage/Learning Matters.

CHAPTER 5
GATHERING AND ANALYSING INFORMATION

This chapter will introduce you to the important skills associated with gathering and analysing information in order to write effective assignments and make effective decisions in practice settings. To be successful in assignment writing you will need to develop skills of reflection and analysis (see Chapters 3 and 4). We hope this chapter will help you to develop confidence in gathering and analysing information. We include extracts from real assignments and we will introduce you to useful tools to use for analysing information.

There is an expectation whilst undertaking the degree that students not only read a great deal of literature but also make judgements about it in order to best apply the learning to social work practice.

THIS CHAPTER WILL HELP YOU TO:

1   Search for literature to draw on in assignments.
2   Develop skills in analysing information from a range of sources.
3   Use a range of tools for analysing information and consider how to apply these skills in assignments.
4   Develop an awareness of the importance of research-mindedness in social work.

Our advice to you is to develop a questioning approach to sources of information, to take nothing at face value, and question not only *what* is being said but also *who* is saying it. As in popular detective novels and detective TV programmes, things may not be as they seem on the surface; the evidence has to be gathered, sifted, analysed and prioritised in order to determine a pattern and a solution and there may be false trails and misleading clues.

We will use extracts from actual student assignments to illustrate some of the points made in this chapter.

The Benchmarks for Social Work

What is expected on completion of the qualifying social work award is set out clearly in the Benchmarks for Social Work (QAA 2008). Gathering and analysing information is fundamental to the role of a social worker, and the range of skills involved are listed in a section of the Benchmarks in a section which focusses on gathering information.

'On completion of the degree you should be able to

- gather information from a wide range of sources and by a variety of methods, for a range of purposes. These methods should include electronic searches, reviews of relevant literature, policy and procedures, face-to-face interviews, written and telephone contact with individuals and groups
- take into account differences of viewpoint in gathering information and
- critically assess the reliability and relevance of the information gathered
- assimilate and disseminate relevant information in reports and case records'.

(QAA 2008: 5.5.2)

The Benchmark document also include a list of statements in relation to analysis and synthesis, with this list emphasising the applied nature of the social work qualifying programme and the rationale for learning this set of skills.

'By the end of the programme of study you should be able to

- analyse information gathered, weighing competing evidence and modifying their point in light of new information, then relate this information to a particular task, situation or problem
- consider specific factors relevant to social work practice (such as risk, rights, cultural differences and linguistic sensitivities, responsibilities to protect vulnerable individuals and legal obligations)
- assess the merits of contrasting theories, explanations, research, policies and procedures
- synthesise knowledge and sustain reasoned argument
- employ a critical understanding of human agency at the macro (societal), mezzo(organisational and community) and micro (inter and intrapersonal) levels
- critically analyse and take account of the impact of inequality and discrimination in work with people in particular contexts and problem situations'.

(QAA 2008: 5.5.3)

The Professional Capability Framework for social work (College of Social Work 2012a) sets out the capabilities in relation to knowledge, skills and values that you are expected to demonstrate at different stages of a social worker's career.

In the domain of *critical reflection* at the level of readiness for direct practice this involves

- 'understanding the need to construct hypotheses in social work practice' and
- being able to 'recognise and describe why evidence is important in social work practice'.

By the end of first placement you should be able to:

- 'recognise the importance of applying imagination, creativity and curiosity to practice
- inform decision-making through the identification and gathering of information from more than one source and, with support, question its reliability and validity
- with guidance understand how to evaluate and review hypotheses in response to information available at the time and apply in practice with support and with guidance use evidence to inform decisions'.

On completion of the final placement you should be able to:

- apply imagination, creativity and curiosity to practice;
- inform decision-making through the identification and gathering of information from multiple sources, actively seeking new sources;
- support, rigorously question and evaluate the reliability and validity of information from different sources;
- demonstrate a capacity for logical, systematic, critical and reflective reasoning and apply the theories and techniques of reflective practice;
- know how to formulate, test, evaluate and review hypotheses in response to information available at the time and apply in practice;
- begin to formulate and make explicit, evidence-informed judgements and justifiable decisions.

The social work programme you are enrolled in will incorporate all of these in its design, and, through participating in the teaching and learning activities and successfully completing the assignments and practice learning placements, you will be able to demonstrate your achievement of them.

5.1 HOW TO SEARCH FOR INFORMATION

A wide range of information from a wide range of sources can be used to inform social work practice. You will have access to the extensive resources of the university library, in both physical and electronic forms, and will be provided with guidance in order to access them, both on and off campus. In addition to the traditional library resources of books and peer-reviewed journals, there are other sources of information to consider in order to develop insights into the experiences of service users and carers. Arts and humanities materials, such as films, poetry, drama and narrative accounts can provide an enriching and creative learning experience (Pulman et al. 2012, Quinney et al. 2012) and access to a wider spectrum of evidence that can be used to guide practice.

Example

As part of a unit/module entitled 'Exploring Evidence to Guide Practice' students are introduced to a triangular model to understand the experiences of the people they will be working with in practice settings. The three points of the triangle represent: first-person accounts; technical knowledge and research evidence; and personal and life resources. These can also be considered to represent a merging of social work values, knowledge and skills, including the important concept of *use of self*, see Fig. 5.1.

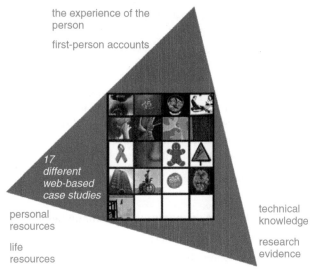

FIGURE 5.1 The unit/module philosophy.

Social work students consider narrative accounts of the experience of parental substance misuse, watching clips from YouTube produced by the Children's Society, watching excerpts from a television documentary aimed at children accessed from the *Box of Broadcasting* facility, and reading a poem written by a child whose parent misuses alcohol, taken from a research report. They read a selection of research papers into the experience of parental substance misuse which use a range of methodological approaches, and consider policy documents. Podcasts by the module team about research methodology are also available. By critically reflecting on this range of material students evaluate its application to practice. Students commented on the value of this service user-focussed way of learning about research.

The narrative material 'was really valuable in focussing my perceptions and assumptions and is something I will realise the importance of in practice. I also feel that I have learnt how important it is to do research, particularly in practice, as it really helps to inform what you do and challenge in the workplace'.

'Being able to read papers and listen to podcasts helped me have a deeper understanding about individuals and their life experiences. It's given me greater imagination and insight into what evidence based practice is all about'.

(Pullman et al., 2012)

TOP TIP   Tips for identifying relevant sources

- Avoid literature aimed at pre-university level. Whilst these texts can be useful to gain a very basic understanding of a subject, it is advisable not to rely on this material when writing academic assignments.
- When searching online check the material is up to date, balanced and about social work in the UK, unless you are explicitly considering material from other countries.
- Be cautious if something is not peer-reviewed or published by a recognised publisher.
- Introductory social work texts are useful to develop an understanding of a subject during the early stages of the programme but should not be relied on as you progress through the levels of the programme.
- Be guided by the reading list for the module you are studying.

In our experience students are unclear about which books to buy and which to borrow from the library. Your lecturers may indicate on the reading list the texts that are essential, recommended, or supplementary. Ornstein (1994 in Green Lister 2012) offers a list of criteria for social work educators to consider before recommending textbooks to students. It would be useful for you to consider this list too in order to make decisions about books:

- Is the text up to date and accurate?
- Is it comprehensive?
- Does it adequately and properly portray minority ethnic communities and women?
- Are the objectives, headings and summaries clear?
- Are the contents and index well organised?
- What are the outstanding features of the text?

As well as identifying the textbooks most relevant to the level of study, it is important to learn how to distinguish between different types of textbooks, and how to reference the material in them accurately and using the university referencing format.

- Introductory texts are often summaries of and commentaries on other people's specialist publications.
- An edited textbook offers the opportunity to read chapters written by people who are seen as specialists in that area, for example the popular set of three textbooks edited by professors Robert Adams, Lena Dominelli and Malcolm Payne (Adams et al. 2002, 2005, 2009) This 'trilogy' contains selection of chapters broadly aimed at different levels of the social work degree programme.
- A single authored textbook has been written by one author. This might be someone who is seen as a specialist in a particular area. An example are the textbooks on social work skills by Pam Trevithick, the latest issue being Trevithick (2012).
- A multi-authored text book has been written by several authors who have shared the responsibility for all the material, such as this one or the extensive introductory text by Wilson et al. (2011). In this latter example additional material was provided by specialist authors.

It is important to read or buy the most recent edition as the legal and policy context of social work changes rapidly and later editions also draw on the most recent new research. If you have been recommended to read a 'classic' text, you will need to be aware of the changes over time in the field of social work.

We emphasise consistently throughout this book that the process of social work education will not equip you with simple answers to complex situations, rather it stimulates critical thought and problem solving. This is equally true with textbooks. Crisp et al. (2006 in Green Lister 2012) argue that introductory sociology books, for example, socialise students to a discipline. It is important to then move on to reading texts by the specialist thinkers and writers. An author may favour a particular school of thought or approach and advocate this within the text. This can feel confusing, as it gives the impression that the author is offering an 'answer' when, as we have already established, there are no simple 'correct' answers in social work. Green Lister (2012) insightfully highlights further concerns surrounding what is known as 'mentioning'. This, she suggests, occurs in textbooks which try to be too comprehensive, and so offer only a superficial mention or consideration of a subject.

When reading a textbook you should therefore be aware of the following points:

- When it was written.
- Whether it offers an in-depth account of a subject.
- Whether it only offers one or several potential solution/theory/intervention etc.

And ask:

- Does it comprehensively tackle a subject?
- Is it supported by evidence?
- Is there external evidence which supports/challenges its statements?
- The audience it is intended for (level of study).

TAKE A MOMENT TO REFLECT ...

Think about this book. Were you attracted to it because it is written by an experienced social work lecturer with a keen interest in how students learn and recent social work graduates who are practising social workers, from their perspective as students? Did you consider the authors to be as important, or less important than the subject matter? Or was your choice based on a combination of the two?

5.1.1 Literature searches

Your university library service will be able to provide you with information about undertaking literature searches using the library resources. Your university will have subscriptions to a broad range of peer-reviewed social work journals which will be searchable using databases. Your search may be undertaken using author name or keywords. You may need to register for a password in order to access resources.

 TOP TIP

As you will be using the internet to access resources for your assignments, we recommend that you develop and practise information searching skills. We have identified a useful online tutorial in the *Further reading* section at the end of the chapter, designed to help you search for social work literature.

5.1.2 Literature reviews

Once you have gathered material from undertaking a literature search, you will then need to sift through and organise the material, making judgements about its usefulness for the particular assignment you are working on. You may be asked to write a literature review as an assignment in its own right, perhaps as part of a proposal for a dissertation or extended study, and the process of producing a literature review is a sound basis for all assignments. The purpose of the literature review is to identify the key messages, themes and issues – and the gaps – in a topic area.

A thorough review will include the following:

- Identify and analyse what research has been undertaken and what the findings were.
- Identify what other material has been written on the topic – this might uncover the relevant government policy priorities and, in the context of this assignment, the current practice priorities.

It is important to be aware of the service user and carer perspective – please ensure you include sources that address this.

The review should be thorough and purposeful, based on an effective literature search of university databases, rather than an ad hoc search using Google or similar. You will have access to an enormous amount of material using the university library as a gateway.

According to Hart (1998: 1) the literature review should have 'appropriate breadth and depth, rigour and consistency, clarity and brevity, and effective analysis and synthesis'. The review combines library and computer skills with intellectual skills of analysis and synthesis – involving finding the right literature and assessing the value of the literature.

The purposes of the literature review include:

- Distinguishing what has been done from what needs to be done.
- Discovering important variables relevant to the topic.
- Synthesising and gaining a new perspective.
- Identifying relationships between ideas and practice.
- Establishing the context of the topic or problem.
- Rationalising the significance of the problem.
- Enhancing and acquiring the subject vocabulary.
- Understanding the structure of the subject.
- Relating ideas and theory to applications.
- Identifying the methodologies and techniques used.
- Understanding the historical context and current situation.
- Distinguishing what has been done from what needs to be done.
- Discovering important variables relevant to the topic.
- Synthesising and gaining a new perspective.
- Identifying relationships between ideas and practice.
- Establishing the context of the topic or problem.
- Rationalising the significance of the problem.
- Enhancing and acquiring the subject vocabulary.
- Understanding the structure of the subject.
- Relating ideas and theory to applications.
- Identifying the methodologies and techniques used.
- Understanding the historical context and current situation.

5.2 HOW TO ANALYSE INFORMATION

As you have seen, reviewing the literature on a given topic involves analysis of the material in order to determine its relevance. During the social work degree you will come across the term *postmodernism*. Postmodernism is an approach which seeks to offer an understanding of how knowledge is created. It seeks to analyse not only the knowledge itself but also who is making the claims about the development of knowledge. Jan Fook (2002), an internationally known and respected social work author, states that postmodern and critical thinkers challenge traditional ideas of knowledge in a number of ways:

- By asking what constitutes acceptable knowledge and whether and why some forms of knowledge are valued over others.
- By focussing on how we know, as well as what we know.
- By drawing attention to different perspectives on what and how we know.
- By drawing attention to the perspectives of the knower, and how it influences what is known and how it is known.

Remember, knowledge is not absolute. What we know now will differ from what we thought we knew previously, and no doubt it will differ from what we will know in the future. By applying the points raised by Jan Fook we can begin to analyse not only the claims to knowledge but also why those claims are being made and by whom. This in turn enables us to 'authenticate' information.

5.2.1 Thinking about information differently

A world where social work students and social worker practitioners could implicitly trust all sources of information would most likely be less complicated and less stressful. However, this utopian world does not exist and social work does not operate in an idealistic vacuum. Rather, it operates within a complex system of human relationships and societal influences, whilst simultaneously balancing financial constraints and a heavily bureaucratic system.

It is essential that you begin to develop your analytical skills whilst in a safe academic environment, as these skills will be essential for your ethical decision making within fieldwork. We have worked alongside successful students who do not take information at face value, who have learnt to ask questions such as: who are the authors? What are their backgrounds? What makes their view on social work any more relevant than other writers or that of the people who receive services? Where is the information derived from? We strongly recommend that you adopt a curious, questioning and analytical stance to maximise your learning. In the contested area of social work there are always arguments and counter-arguments to consider, there are always areas which require further analysis. Just like a detective, you must develop a 'quizzical' approach to information and gather as many sources as possible to validate an argument.

5.3 TOOLS FOR ANALYSING INFORMATION AND APPLYING THEM IN ASSIGNMENTS

Effectively analysing information involves:

- Examining information from a number of different angles.
- Comparing the same issue from different points of view.
- Being able to understand why people arrive at different conclusions.

- Recognising inaccuracies or gaps.
- Being able to argue why one conclusion is preferable to another.
- Recognising hidden assumptions or possible flaws in reasoning or conclusions.
- Being aware of indicators of validity.

It is a skill that you should develop as your learning progresses – it is both an academic skill and an essential social work practice skill. Developing this skill whilst studying will enhance your sound ethical decision making once in practice, as practitioners are often presented with vast amounts of information which require well-developed analytical skills to ensure the information presented is utilised effectively and appropriately for the benefit of service users and carers.

5.3.1 Checklist 1

Critical questions	Analysis of the writing
1. What is the main line of reasoning or argument? 2. Is the main line of reasoning clear throughout? 3. What is the key evidence used to support the line of argument? Is the evidence presented in a way that develops the argument and leads clearly to the conclusion? 4. When was the evidence produced? Is it still up to date and relevant? 5. Is there sufficient evidence to justify the findings? What might be missing? 6. Are there any examples of flawed reasoning or any attempts to persuade the reader through an appeal to emotions? Is the evidence interpreted and used correctly? 7. Has the writer given sufficient consideration to alternative views? Give examples. 8. Check for transparency. Has the author made attempts to highlight any conflicts of interests or ethical issues? Can you see any hidden messages? 9. Who has published the material? Could they have anything to gain from its publication? 10. Does the writer consider/utilise the service user perspective? 11. Are the practice implications clear?	

(Adapted from Cottrell 2011)

This can be used when reading textbooks, journal articles or research reports.

When considering the points in the table, you are trying to ascertain whether the evidence is sound. Do you consider that the information presented is inclusive or selective? Consider the date of the publication or of the research project; whilst 'old' research may be useful it is important is that you find the most up-to-date research possible. Deciding on the sufficiency and completeness of the information requires further reading around the subject to ascertain whether other authors or studies support or challenge the ideas or the findings.

Has the author included information about the size of the study and adequate information about how they undertook their research? Compare their findings with their concluding remarks, for example, when 51% of people said they liked their social worker to always wear sandals, has the author used words such as 'the majority of people' (which could be considered misleading) or 'People reported that they preferred sandal-wearing social workers' (this too is ambiguous). Ensure findings and concluding statements are congruent.

Consider how sound the reasoning is. For example, flawed reasoning occurs when an assumption is made that two incidents must be connected in some way. Consider whether there might be other possible factors which could influence the findings or provide alternative perspectives. Emotive language can be very persuasive, leading the reader to place trust in what they are reading. Emotive words such as 'extreme', 'abuse', 'natural', 'cruel', or 'normal' can prompt emotional responses that may lead the reader away from an accurate appraisal of the evidence. Persuasive words such as 'obviously', 'clearly', 'it is evident that', or 'absolutely' draw the reader in by appealing to what they claim is clear evidence. The use of persuasive words does not necessarily mean that the findings are inaccurate but you should nevertheless be aware of them. Consider whether the author has given sufficient consideration to alternative views. This will involve you reading around the subject to identify any alterative views.

Are there any conflicts of interests, if so are they clearly identified? Have all ethical issues been considered and has the research received ethical approval? Has the writer sought service users' views if appropriate? If not consider why not. If they have, does the writer inclusively and clearly detail the service user perspective?

5.3.2 Checklist 2

Another useful framework for analysing information is offered by Pawson et al. (2003) published by the Social Care Institute for Excellence. The authors acknowledge that this model does not necessarily identify 'good' knowledge, but it helps practitioners and students to identify weakness in information. When reading any form of literature you can ask yourself 'is this TAPUPAS?': that is, does it meet the standards identified below?

Transparency

Accuracy

Purposivity

Utility

Propriety

Accessibility

Transparency – are the reasons for it clear? Is the knowledge open to outside scrutiny? To be able to meet this standard it should be made clear how the knowledge was generated, identifying what steps the author has gone through to give the reader an understanding of the argument.

Questions you may ask:

- How has the author come to this conclusion?
- Are full details given about how the study was conducted?
- Does the author identify any possible flaws?
- Does the author give clear reasons why the study has been conducted?
- Does the author identify who funded the study?
- Does the author make any conflicts of interests clear?

Extract from a student assignment

Both studies in this assignment state who commissioned the research allowing the reader to draw their own conclusions regarding any bias. Lloyd and Clarke's (2002) research was commissioned and published by the Men's Health Forum which describes itself 'as the leading voluntary organisation promoting a gender-sensitive approach to health' (MHF 2007). The forum states that men 'do worse in many areas of health', providing a perspective from which to reflect upon the recommendations made.

Accuracy – is it honestly based on relevant evidence? All knowledge claims should be supported by the events, experiences, informants and sources used in their production. All recommendations, assertions or conclusion should be based on an honest account of material and information gathered.

Questions you may ask:

- Is the study supported by independent sources?
- If service users views are being sought are they asserted or are their views and experiences detailed within the study?
- If the study analyses/utilises existing information is this selective or all-inclusive?
- Is there any information which has been omitted? Has a rationale been offered to explain this?

> ### Extract from a student assignment
>
> *Having considered the implications of any bias in the studies undertaken by Lloyd & Clarke (2002) and Pinfold (2003) I believe that the authors of the former research study present stronger argument to underpin their findings. Despite a relatively small number of participants, the researchers have captured the feelings of the young men involved, providing insights into the difficulties of engaging with this group. Furthermore, the researchers give examples of good practice for policy makers and practitioners to build upon.*

Purposivity – is the method used suitable for the aims of the work? The approaches used to gather data/create knowledge should be fit for purpose and appropriate for the task. For knowledge to meet this standard it should demonstrate that the enquiry has followed the opposite approach to meet the stated objective of the exercise.

Questions you may ask:

- What methods have been used to gain the knowledge?
- How have the research team ensured the study is 'fit for purpose' - is the right question being asked in the right way, to the right people?

> ### Extract from a student assignment
>
> *The DoH (2006) illustrated purposivity through their careful planning of the research. The planning phase lasted six months to ensure the research would be 'fit for purpose'. The research team carefully considered how they achieved each objective including process planning, formation of the team, training for research mindedness, preparation of interview questions and compilation of a research pack. In contrast, although the research study by McGlaughlin et al. (2004) appears 'fit for purpose', a possible weakness of the study is the elimination of people who the researchers deemed to be 'inappropriate for inclusion'. People who had recently experienced a housing crisis were considered to be too vulnerable to interview. Whilst this might be seen as demonstrating sensitivity to individuals, it could also be considered a limitation of the study as these voices are not heard.*

Utility – does it provide answers to the questions it set? The knowledge should be appropriate to the setting/subject in which it is being used. For knowledge to meet this standard, it needs to be fit for use and provide answers that are as closely matched as possible to the question. For example, practitioners looking for knowledge on how to help first-generation immigrant families experiencing alcohol-related problems may consider not only information about the disorder but also information sensitive to the background, history, culture and context of the client.

Questions you may ask:

- Have the most appropriate individuals' views been sought?
- Have the most appropriate methods been used to collect data?
- Has the question been answered?

Extract from a student assignment

The groundbreaking nature of the DoH (2006) research, combined with its utility for policy makers across the UK means that it could have a significant impact on increased opportunities for people with a learning disability to fully participate in future research projects.

Propriety – is it legal and ethical? Knowledge should be created legally, ethically and with due care to all relevant stakeholders. For knowledge to meet this standard, it should present adequate evidence, appropriate to each point of contact, of the informed consent of relevant stakeholders.

Questions you may ask:

- Has the study received ethical approval?
- Has consent been gained from each stakeholder?
- Has information that has been withheld also received consent from the individual who has offered it?

Extract from a student assignment

Both studies considered informed consent, accurate evidence, and the DoH (2006) research provided copies of the research to all participants to ensure they met the standard of propriety.

Accessibility – can you understand it? Knowledge should be presented in a way that is accessible to the seeker of that information. To meet this standard no potential seeker of information should be excluded to accessing or reading it based purely on how the information is presented.

Questions you may ask:

- Is it understandable to the target audience?
- Is it culturally sensitive to the target audience – i.e. is it written in the appropriate language?
- Does it use professional terminology appropriately (this will depend on who the target audience is)?
- How is the information disseminated – does this enable access for its target audience?

> **Extract from a student assignment**
>
> *Both studies are written in a style which is free from medical or scientific jargon aimed at maximising their multi-disciplinary appeal. Lloyd and Clarke's (2002) paper is written in an accessible style reflecting the authors' values on inclusion and equality.*

An additional word, Specificity, was later added to TAPUPA, to become TAPUPAS.

Specificity – does it meet the quality standards already used for this type of knowledge? Questions you may ask:

- Is it disseminated within a peer-reviewed journal?
- Is it disseminated within a journal appropriate to the studies' content?
- Has it been subject to the normal rigorous testing of peer-reviewed journals? Has this been made explicit within the study?

ACTIVITY 1A

In order to recap on what you have learnt so far, make some notes on why you need to develop skills in gathering and analysing information.

ACTIVITY 1B

What could happen if students/social workers do not check the accuracy or validity of information or make assumptions?

A student's response to Activity 1a

I need to develop these skills as part of my academic work in order to be a better practitioner. For me, getting it right for service users is the core component of my aspiration to be a social worker. To achieve this I need specific information gathering and analysing skills to apply in my practice. Firstly, I need to be able to make sense of the presenting information contained in a referral. I need to consider the information provided and make judgements about priorities and risks and consider what further information I need to gather. Next I need planning skills, to ensure I am fully prepared for beginning an interaction or intervention. I need to weigh up whether I understood the problem from the service users' perspective and consider other professionals who might be involved – have I made any assumptions and have I explained my role and remit?

Developing and refining these skills will help me to build effective partnerships with service users and colleagues.

A student's response to Activity 1b

I remember one example where a referral about an elderly man in residential care went wrong in a number of ways.

The referral contained information about the safety and welfare of the man. The duty officer talked to his relative who said they did not want to make a complaint or cause a problem. The recommended course of action was noted as a social work review rather than an adult protection investigation. For three weeks the case was unallocated due to staff shortages and low priority. When finally allocated the social worker assumed it was not serious as nothing had been done. When the social worker reviewed the elderly man's placement she found he had experienced neglect. He had memory loss, was not able to express his needs and was reliant on the support of others to ensure his health and welfare was maintained.

The social workers involved were trying to weigh up need and risk against ever-increasing scarcity of resources. Clearer exploration of the situation and information gathering at the referral stage could have revealed the alleged neglect, despite the relative's desire not to be seen as a 'complainer'. This could have minimised the distress experienced by the elderly man. I can't think of a better reason for getting clear and accurate information in order to make a decision.

ACTIVITY 2

Can you think of any situations where you have questioned information? You may want to consider:

- News stories in newspapers, news websites and news programmes
- Government reports
- Advertising.

We will use the example of the highly publicised and emotive public sector strikes of 2011 and 2012 which drew a range of strong and often opposing views. Here we present two opposing perspectives on this issue.

Conservative MP Dominic Raab was reported as saying:

As the country grapples with a serious debt crisis, union leaders wreaked havoc by inflicting on Britain the most working days lost to strikes since the poll tax. With the overwhelming majority of strikes failing to win support from a majority of union members, it demonstrates the arbitrary power wielded by union bosses. It is time we looked seriously at the case for reform, to safeguard the hard-working majority from the militant minority.

(Telegraph 2012)

However, the Unison stance on the strikes differed, with trade unionists presenting the following statistics and arguments.

- Mortgages up 8%
- Petrol up 22%
- Bread up 9%
- Milk up 17%
- Fuel bills up 15%
- Inflation up 4.3%

But council workers are being offered a pay rise of just 2.45%. Take inflation into account and it's a pay CUT. That's why hundreds of thousands of our members stood together to take action in July. The services our members provide are essential to local communities. And unless we get a fair settlement, those communities will suffer. Services will simply get worse as councils continue to lose committed staff and struggle to find new employees prepared to work for such low pay and poor conditions. We empty your bins, clean your schools, conduct your marriages and civil partnerships, care for your parks, check the safety of your food and look after your children in nurseries, schools and in care. And so much more. In exchange, all we are asking for is your support for a fair deal.

(Unison 2012)

One very complicated issue but two very different stances that offer seemingly equally 'sensible' arguments, backed up with claims of evidence.

Looking back on what you have read so far in this chapter, what might help you make sense of this news item in order not to accept these arguments at face value? What questions might you ask?

5.3.3 Extracts from student assignments

We have included some further assignment extracts to illustrate how students have approached the use of analysis of material in their assignments.

Example 1

In this assignment the student attempts to demonstrate their awareness and understanding of the value of evidence-based practice. This approach involves social workers using knowledge which has been gathered and tested empirically in the most rigorous ways possible, to inform actions which are most likely to achieve a particular objective.

For example, a Canadian study using focus groups identify the theme 'suffering in silence' (Walsh et al. 2007: 492) which shows the reluctance of older people to talk about familial abuse due to fear of retaliation, shame and embarrassment, or 'for the love of their children'. The study confirmed previous research findings that older women are more likely to be abused than older men (Fulmer et al. 2004; Straka and Montminy 2006). Whilst Zink et al. (2003) believe this is the result of older women being more likely to be socialised to be submissive, Rennison and Rand (2003) argue that other generational factors such as traditional gender roles, attitudes towards marriage, plus the fear of being alone make it more likely that older women will stay in an abusive relationship.

Example 2

The student in this example has used the notion of social construction. Payne (2005) argues that knowledge and understanding of the world comes from social interactions amongst people. He suggests that a useful aspect of social construction is its distinct approach to research. Analysing video and audio tape of human interaction enables supporters of this approach to reveal patterns of communication and behaviour which may have previously been hidden. Social construction engages people who are subject to research in an equal relationship with the researcher. The aim here is to explore situations from many different angles consequently producing a fuller picture of complex human situations.

Reflecting on the simulated video conference I observed gestures of displacement and anxiety, manifested in fiddling with a pen and hand rings when imparting sensitive information to the client. Two individuals presented with submissive or defensive body language evidenced by their body position and stiffly closed arms and legs. Both students' facial expressions captured my interest; the first with nervy, darting eye contact that sought acceptance and reassurance, the second appearing to 'grimace' perhaps indicating discomfiture in role play as Goffman's (1959) theory of impression management suggests how embarrassment or 'invalidation of role' results in performance breakdown. Another student appeared impatient to ask a great deal of questions to the detriment of collaboration and listening to others, which Tuckman (1977) identifies as an attempt to establish identity or leadership within the group. This 'jostling' for position was evident in a number of participants.

Example 3

In this example the student was focussing on the notion of empowerment, which give spriority to the wishes of service users. Since they are often oppressed, disadvantaged and marginalised, supporters of the empowerment view argue that the service users' understanding of their situation should be what guides social work practice. Empowerment views argue that service users often have the best knowledge of their circumstances and objectives, which should therefore be followed.

> *'Let me in, I'm a researcher' (DoH 2006) was a groundbreaking study as adults with a learning disability managed and undertook the research. The study considered its oppressive potential and made practice decisions to ensure participants felt empowered. They published a project leaflet, the appendix reproduced the full questionnaire, and the report provided a level of detail that would ensure the study could be replicated. The research was accessible to interested readers through its use of pictures, simple summaries and bullet points. One noteworthy aspect was the attention to diversity within the research team and the apparent value for individual skills and contributions. The team reported on their planning phase to ensure the research would be 'fit for purpose'. This included training on research-mindedness, preparation of the interview questions and the development of a research pack for the use of researchers. Furthermore the DoH research provided copies of the study to all participants to ensure they met the standard of propriety. Importantly, the research group was considered by DoH as a professional group and remunerated accordingly. This study appears to attempt a shift in organisational rigorous research beliefs by embracing core Valuing People principles of respect, promoting social justice and addressing inequality.*

However, empowerment, whilst a cornerstone of social work practice, also presents practitioners with tensions and dilemmas, as this second year student explores.

> *The ideology of self-determination is well documented in social work literature (Payne 1997, Pritchard 1999) and echoed by GSCC (2002) who stress that the basic principle of good practice is self-determination and the right of competent adults to take risks and refuse intervention. Preston Shoot and Wigley (2002) consider these principles by analysing effective practice under No Secrets (DoH 2000). The research provides examples of failure of practitioners to act even where there was clear evidence of abuse as it was against the victim's wishes. It appears that many social workers privileged self-determination over protection even when the person was confused (Preston-Shoot and Wigley 2002). The study highlighted that the procedures did not provide guidance to practitioners in such circumstances, leaving this to professional judgements undertaken by risk assessment which by its very nature is subject to the bias of one's value base. The Mental Capacity Act 2005 now provides a safeguard for the protection of vulnerable adults through the formal testing of mental capacity. This means that the 'best interests' of people deemed as lacking capacity are safeguarded, and professional 'neglect' is now viewed as a criminal offence and subject to police investigation and prosecution. However, in my experience adult protection remains a problematic area of social work where vulnerable adults, deemed to have capacity, make decisions that others may view as unwise or risky. Wilson (1994) cautions against failing to take the imbalance of power in an ageist and patriarchal society into consideration when reflecting on the conflicting ideologies of empowerment versus protection which may prevent people from accepting help; for example the victim may rely on the alleged abuser for their care. This, according to Preston-Shoot (2002), suggests that self-determination alone may be problematic as the sole guiding principle for elder adult protection social work.*

Example 4

In this example the student is considering realist views which argue that knowledge emerges from human interpretations of successions of events that can be captured empirically. Realist proponents argue that social phenomena exist beyond social constructions but that the constructions are nevertheless important to understand. Often described as critical realism, this approach utilises both an evidence-based and social construction view.

Lloyd et al. (2002) approached the argument by the posing of two questions; namely whether in fact social workers do experience greater stress than other health colleagues, and if so, what factors contribute to their stress and burnout. Lloyd (2002) alludes to a complex psychological confusion arising from unclear aims and objectives that resulted in lowered self-esteem, confidence and motivation, and argues that social work burnout was closely associated with the experiences of such emotions. Moreover, Lloyd (2002) proposes that a susceptibility to stress is inevitable due to social workers' innate sensitivity to others problems, and Acker (1999) supports this claim, arguing that that the nature of social work attracts candidates whose personality traits might predispose them to stress-related feelings and emotions. Collins (2007) lends credence to this view, indicating a correlation between personality and vulnerability to stress. However, Jones (2001) believes that individual knowledge, ability and perception of control experienced in changing cultural and structural climates could be a more prevailing factor, invoking powerful negative emotions at a personal level. Jones' evocative and stark 2001 study concluded that a climate of fear and an ideology of managerialism led to a culture of 'blame' which has fragmented social work practice.

Example 5

In this assignment the student demonstrates their awareness and understanding of the process of research in order to make judgements about the potential application of the studies they have read to their future practice.

Both studies are examples of qualitative research which attempts to gain in-depth opinion from participants by exploring attitudes, behaviour and experiences through methods such as interviews and focus groups (Bell 1999). Pinfold's (2003) paper is explicit from the outset that the research was jointly commissioned by the NHS and DoH. The author states that Rethink currently operate 13 helplines funded by the NHS or jointly with local authorities, information which allows the reader to identify potential bias and consider the findings accordingly. Pinfold's (2003) study involved a small sample and the lack of feedback from the service users themselves meant the findings rely on the opinions of internal and external stakeholders. Whilst this is a valid approach it did not offer the same insight into alternative models of good practice as Lloyd and Clarke (2003). A further criticism of the research is that despite small numbers to deal with, Pinfold (2003) does not indicate the participants' gender, age or ethnicity, which may have been valuable in terms of service development. In contrast, the paper by Lloyd and Clarke (2003) examines the diversity of their participant group comprehensibly. The potential for transferability of these findings is clearer and the authors attempt to identify good models of practice with diverse groups and communities.

We can see from these assignment extracts that there are many different ways of interpreting literature and situations. We will introduce you to the value of becoming a research-minded practitioner in the following section.

5.4 BECOMING A RESEARCH-MINDED PRACTITIONER

This involves the ability to access research, evaluate research findings and apply them to practice situations. It has been defined in the following way (Centre for Human Services Technology 2005):

- an ability to engage in critical reflection about practice that is informed by professional knowledge and research;

- an ability to use research to inform practice which seeks to challenge unfair discrimination, racism, poverty, disadvantage and injustice, consistent with core professional values;

- an understanding of the process of research and the use of research to theorise from practice.

You may come across a range of terms including research-based practice, evidence-based practice, research-informed practice but here we will use the term research-mindedness.

During the social work degree programme you will be learning about the process of research in order to raise your awareness of its potential to inform practice, and at master's level you may be required to undertake a small-scale research project of your own. In a research study into how students develop confidence in accessing, understanding and applying research skills it was felt important that 'being able to engage with research will enable practitioners to develop practice based on competent reading of research and contribute to the enhancement of the profession and its research base' (Quinney and Parker 2010: 17).

In a study for the Social Care Institute for Excellence, Fisher and Marsh (2005) clearly set out the value of research for practice.

1. Decisions made by practitioners can have an immediate impact on people's lives so having the best informed practitioners is vital to the immediate outcomes for highly disadvantaged people (by health or circumstances).

2. Over time, decisions can have an important impact on life chances of patients, service users and carers.

3. Research findings can inform the development of new policies that enhance people's life chances.

4. Research can provide safeguards where the state has compulsory powers by helping us understand the decision-making process and providing evidence for those decisions.

5. Members of the public are able to participate in the debates about future policy and practice if they are informed by having access to research evidence.

6. Patients, service users and carers have access to some research evidence and expect to be involved in decisions and debates about service delivery and service development.

Research helps us understand decision-making processes and provide a rationale for the decisions made, for example on educational outcomes of looked-after children or on the outcomes for people with a mental health diagnosis. Research on personalisation has promoted a shift in the balance of power in the way in which services are provided. Accessible research can facilitate public participation in debates, for example the proposed changes to paying for care, which will have an impact on us all in the future. Service users have a voice through organisations and pressure groups such as Age Concern, Mind, the Alzheimer's Society, and the dissemination of research should be in a range of formats for a range of audiences (e.g. Dr Kip Jones' work *Rufus Stone the movie*).

Not only does research need to be meaningful to practitioners, but it also needs to be readily available and accessible. Much research is published in peer-reviewed journals, requiring a subscription, and whilst we encourage the use of peer-reviewed academic journals you may not have the facilities of a university library when you are no longer a student. There are other sources of research material, for example the repository of the Social Care Institute for Excellence (www.scie.org.uk) and the Joseph Rowntree Foundation (www.jrf.org.uk). It is important to become aware of research institutions that disseminate research and of the host universities of key names where their research may be available on public areas of university websites. An example is the Tilda Goldberg research centre at the University of Bedfordshire which is undertaking a body of work into substance misuse and the impact on families.

Importantly, practitioners need to be motivated and able to access research. Demystifying the research process can encourage future practitioners to become not only research-minded but also research active and to share in the process of developing social work services. Research needs to be meaningful and reflect the issues facing practitioners and service users.

Practitioners need to have the motivation, the means and the time to access, evaluate and apply research findings and to be active participants in learning in the workplace (Walter et al. 2004). Critical evaluation of the research is important in order to determine its utility (usefulness) for the practice situations in which you are involved. Being critical involves reaching new understandings that are more detailed, informed and reasoned by weighing up arguments for and against and looking more closely at what is being said. It involves being sceptical, curious and open to new ideas. This is a good time to revisit the material in Chapter 4 on critical thinking and critical writing.

Not only should research inform practice but it is also important to develop partnerships between researchers and health and care providers in order to ensure that practice informs research – that the concerns of practitioners are informing the research undertaken, and that new knowledge is co-produced. It is vital that research outputs make a difference to those who fund, deliver and receive services. There is a growing body of research involving the co-production of knowledge, with practitioners and researchers collaborating on projects and research with service users and carers as co-researchers.

SELF-ASSESSMENT TOOL

Rate yourself on a scale of 1–10 (10 being the highest) on each of the questions and monitor this over time during the degree programme, and in the future as part of your ongoing professional development and lifelong learning.

1. I understand the importance and relevance of research to practice.
2. I understand the broad principles involved in research.
3. I understand the ethical issues involved in research.
4. I know how to access, understand and summarise research studies.
5. I know how to make use of anti-oppressive perspectives in evaluating research and practice.
6. I know how to identify research which is relevant to practice in which I am involved.
7. I know how to relate research to practice issues and demonstrate how relevant research informs practice.

CONCLUSION

We would like to leave you with the words of Humphries (2008: 3)

'[R]esearch mindedness requires a commitment – even a passion – on the part of practitioners and researchers, which will lead them towards thinking that is beyond common sense, taken-for-granted and instrumental knowledge, where they explore perspectives on social issues that they care deeply about.'

'[A] key ingredient of research-mindedness is a questioning attitude that asks why, and to what purpose.'

We wish you well on your journey to becoming a research-minded practitioner.

FURTHER READING

Carey, M. 2009. *The social work dissertation. Using small scale qualitative methodology.* Maidenhead: McGraw Hill/Open University Press.

Hart, C. 1998. *Doing a literature search.* London: Sage.

McLaughlin, H. 2012. *Understanding social work research.* 2nd ed. London: Sage.

A useful online tutorial to help in developing online searching skills is available from the following address www.vts.intute.ac.uk/tutorial/socialwork/

An online tutorial exploring the importance of being research minded is available from www.resmind.swap.ac.uk

CHAPTER 6
PLANNING AND CONSTRUCTING AN ASSIGNMENT

In this chapter we will consider some common problems in assignment writing and break down assignment writing into steps, illustrating these with extracts from real assignments. It is important that you do not copy these examples as this will constitute plagiarism, an academic offence. Remember, lecturers will be familiar with this chapter too! The extracts are intended to illustrate the points we are making about the process of planning and writing an assignment.

THE CHAPTER WILL COVER THE FOLLOWING AREAS:

1 Some common problems.
2 Understanding the title and intended learning outcomes.
3 Searching for information – how and where to look.
4 Analysing and organising the material.
5 Creating a plan.
6 Developing a clear structure and style.

This chapter builds on the material in the preceding chapters. Having read the previous chapters you should now have a better understanding of some of the fundamental principles of assessment and of the skills underpinning successful academic writing, including reflective writing, critical writing and analysing information. You may want to revisit these chapters alongside working through the guidance we offer in this chapter about the stages of constructing an assignment.

A useful place to start is with a list of questions, developed from Williams (1995).

- **WHAT** do you need to produce? What is the format (for example an essay, report, presentation, portfolio, poster, dissertation or other product)? What does it involve? Remember to check that you understand the assignment guidelines and intended learning outcomes.

- **WHICH** unit is the assignment for? What is the content and focus of that unit? Which lecturer will be marking it?

- **WHY** have you chosen this particular title/topic? What do you want to explore, what puzzles you about a topic or engages your interest, curiosity or passion? What are you hoping to learn?

- **WHEN** is the hand-in date for this assignment – and the other deadlines you are working towards?

- **WHO** will you be working with if this is a group assignment?

- **WHERE** are you likely to find resources?

- **HOW** will you plan and structure your assignment? How will you undertake research and reading? How will you access any support services available to you?

Uncertainty and anxiety about assignments, particularly the first one that you produce as part of your degree course, is not unusual. Williams (1995) suggests that this comes from a desire to produce meaningful and sometimes emotionally difficult material, which is then subject to the judgement of those marking your work. Studying social work involves an emotional engagement with the subject material, particularly when exploring values, ethics and anti-oppressive practice. Working in social work, as well as other areas of health and social care, involves drawing on empathic understanding of the service users' or carers' situation or experience, combined with technical knowledge derived from theory and research and with highly developed practice skills (see Chapter 1). You may feel that it is not only your knowledge that is being judged, but that your beliefs are also being judged and may be anxious about the feedback and the mark you will be awarded. One student may experience the feedback provided as sound practical advice that they will use when constructing future assignments, whereas another may experience the same feedback as devastating and unhelpful. We hope this chapter will help to allay some of these concerns.

There are different expectations at different levels of study and as you progress through the levels of the course you are expected to develop your academic skills to demonstrate your growing understanding, identify the implications for practice through an increased understanding of the relationship between theory and practice whilst providing a consistent and powerful discourse. (You may wish to look back at Chapter 2 to refresh your understanding of the principles and purposes of assessment.)

6.1 SOME COMMON PROBLEMS IN ASSIGNMENTS

Before we start to explore the process of putting together an assignment, it is useful to point out some typical problems in assignments in order for you to be aware of possible pitfalls and avoid them.

- **Not answering the question/addressing the title:** This might include answering only part of the question – if there are two parts to an assignment and you miss out one then it is likely that only 50% of the marks are available. You may have written a very good essay but failed to focus on what was asked of you in the title or question.

- **Not addressing social work values or exploring the implications for social work practice:** Social work is an applied subject and the Social Work Degree provides you with a professional qualification as well as an academic qualification. In order to meet the standards of the profession, you must demonstrate the integration of social work values and make explicit the relationship between theory and practice.

- **Not providing evidence of your own understanding:** This might be through lack of reading and use of key sources, poor referencing, or using too many quotations. It might also be a result of simply rephrasing and restating the material that you have read without demonstrating what this material means in terms of *your* learning for social work practice.

- **Poor structure and organisation:** The structure of your assignment is equally as important as content, as this provides the framework for presenting your understanding of the topic and to drive your arguments.

- **Poor grammar, spelling and punctuation:** These are important skills to master as they are fundamental to clear written communication which is essential in practice settings as well as in academic settings.

- **Writing too much or too little:** It is important to be aware of any word count penalties and make sure you have not exceeded the word count. On some programmes the penalty for exceeding the word count is an automatic fail, on others there are marks deducted depending on the number of excess words. If you submit work that is below the word count, you may not have provided the marker with enough material to demonstrate your understanding.

6.1.1 Poor planning can be a contributory factor

Becoming proficient at accessing, organising, and presenting information is cost-effective. There will be consistent and competing academic pressures to juggle and managing your time well through organisation, and effective planning can help you to more effectively balance study, employment, family time and a social life. It is important not to underestimate the time needed to research, plan and write an assignment, and we strongly recommend avoiding leaving your assignment writing to the night before the hand-in date. It is equally important to maintain a balance between academic work, employment, family time and a social life. Try to build in time for rest and relaxation and to 'recharge your batteries', and to build in time for the unexpected. In case you become ill or experience a family crisis do make sure that you are aware in advance of the university procedures for managing the unexpected impact on your ability to hand in work on time or submitting work that is below your usual standard.

6.1.2 Additional or specific learning needs' assessment, support and equipment

You may already have been identified as having learning needs such as dyslexia, or you may be recommended by programme staff to undertake an assessment. There will normally be additional support available to you, such as one-to-one support in order to develop strategies for learning and for assignment writing. This might include a note-taker in class or additional time for assessments. You may also be eligible for technology equipment or software to support your learning. (There are tips from students who have been diagnosed with dyslexia in Chapter 1.)

6.1.3 Why is developing skills of clear structure, clear arguments and a clear writing style important?

A significant aspect of the social work role involves advocating on behalf of service users and carers, either verbally or in written format. This includes the preparation of assessments and court reports, constructing clear and concise funding requests or emails, presenting information in meetings, and participating in supervision. Persuading people of your argument can involve guiding them through complex information.

6.1.4 What impresses the lecturers marking your assignments?

A study undertaken by Greasley and Cassidy (2009), in a University School of Health and a University School of Social Sciences and Humanities, asked lecturers what they looked for when marking assignments, what impresses them and what frustrates them.

In the study, the **top 10 features that most impressed markers** and had the most positive impact on marks were:

- Critical analysis, perspective and argument (with supporting evidence)
- Following guidelines relating to answering the question and criteria
- Illustrating and applying ideas to specific contexts
- Structure
- Language, grammar and expression
- Reading the relevant literature
- New information (different, original)
- References and referencing
- Introductions and conclusions
- Assimilating feedback.

The **top 10 features that least impressed markers** and had the most negative impact on marks were:

- Failing to answer the question
- Poor language, grammar and expression
- Too much description, too little critical analysis
- Poor structure
- Not following guidelines relating to answering the question and criteria
- Failing to read the relevant literature
- Poor referencing
- Poor introductions and conclusions
- Inappropriate use of quotations
- Poor presentation.

Most of these are equally applicable at both undergraduate and postgraduate levels of study but the comments about critical analysis are particularly relevant as you progress through the levels of the programme on which you are studying.

It is useful to bear these in mind when constructing your assignment, and make a useful checklist when proofreading your work prior to handing it in.

Using this checklist alongside the assignment guidelines will help to improve your marks.

6.2 HOW TO CONSTRUCT AN ASSIGNMENT: UNDERSTANDING THE TITLE/TASK AND THE INTENDED LEARNING OUTCOMES

Do be aware that there is no single approach to constructing an assignment. The steps we set out are general guidelines based on the approaches which have been successfully used by students who have achieved high marks. A good place to start is by clarifying that you understand the title and the intended learning outcomes.

6.2.1 Understanding the title or task

A title can consist of instructions, questions or assertions and needs to be read extremely carefully. It should be read in conjunction with the assignment briefing, checked against the relevant intended learning outcomes for that assessment, in order to ensure you make sound planning decisions. For example, it is usual for all social work assignments to contain a requirement for you to refer to values, to diversity, and to practice implications with an awareness of the experiences of service users and carers.

For illustration we will begin by considering one of the assignment titles from a unit/module on social work with adults. The assignment guidelines state that the essay is 2,000 words in length. You can apply these steps to any assignment you are writing.

Title: Using a community care assessment approach outline and evaluate the key principles underpinning the assessment process outlined in government legislation and national policy documents. Identify any social work theories and values that might influence your assessment. Illustrate your answer with reference to one particular service user group.

Intended learning outcomes:

1. Demonstrate a detailed knowledge of assessment principles and approaches.

2. Identify aspects of the legislative and policy context of social work practice with adults.

3. Present a critical understanding of social work values and service user perspectives.

In addition, it is a requirement of all social work assignments that students demonstrate awareness of anti-discriminatory practice and acknowledge diversity and difference.

The assignment titles you are given will be written in such a way as to enable you to meet the intended learning outcomes.

6.2.2 Step 1 Understanding the task

- Identify the key **content or knowledge words** in **the title** that indicate the areas of knowledge that you have to demonstrate, including the topics, themes, issues and concepts that you are being asked to write about. (You may have highlighted the following – **community care; assessment process; legislation and policy; theories and values.)**

- Note the parameters (limits) set by the question. For example, you are asked to only consider *one* specific service user group. Writing about more than one must be avoided or you will lose marks. You might for example choose adults with a physical disability, adults with dementia, adults with a learning disability, or adults experiencing mental health problems.

- Identify the **action or process words**. For example, in this title you are asked to *evaluate, identify* and *illustrate*.

STOP AND THINK ....

If you are uncertain about the title or the task, it is important to seek clarification from the lecturer involved. Whilst asking other students can be helpful, it is important not to become confused by a range of different interpretations and possibly contradictory information. Use any academic support facilities provided, such as the opportunity to book a tutorial, to email for clarification, information provided on the virtual learning environment (Blackboard, Moodle or a similar system). There may be additional support and guidance offered through a discussion forum, a frequently asked questions bulletin or similar.

6.2.3 Step 2 – a plan of action

Using the content words you have identified make a list of the actions that you will need to undertake in order to write the assignment.

Action or process words

Action or process words	Meaning
Analyse (Analytical)	Examine critically and in detail
Assess (Analytical)	Weigh up
Compare (Analytical)	Find similarities and differences between X and Y
Contrast (Analytical)	Set out the differences
Define (Descriptive)	State the meaning of X; this might involve discovering a range of definitions from different perspectives
Demonstrate	Provide evidence for
Describe (Descriptive)	Provide a detailed account of X
Discuss (Analytical)	Present two or more sides of an argument and their implications
Evaluate (Analytical)	Consider the value or effectiveness of something
Explain	Set out how and why
Identify	Find and present
Illustrate (Descriptive)	Use carefully chosen examples, usually to link theory and practice.
Outline (Descriptive)	Set out the main features
Summarise	A clear account of the main/key aspects of X

(Adapted from Redman and Maples 2011)

In order to answer the question, you will need to do the following:

- identify the key literature in this area and find out about the debates concerning community care assessments;
- choose one service user group and consider the literature specifically in relation to them;
- identify and consider the relative merits of a range of approaches used;
- identify and explore the key principles in the relevant legislation and policy documents – how does this translate into practice; what are the constraints and challenges?
- identify a range of social work theories and values that inform the assessment process.

TAKE A MOMENT TO REFLECT ....

Reflect on your previous assignment writing approaches and what worked best for you. The process of developing assignments is not always linear. You may prefer to tackle different sections in parallel, perhaps starting with the skeleton plan and adding detail in a layering approach, or working in loops and cycles.

6.3 SEARCHING FOR INFORMATION

You will need to undertake a literature search to identify material to read in order to answer the question. The reading list for the unit/module is a good place to start, as are the references in any teaching materials that have been provided on this subject area. You will also need to draw on other relevant material in other units/modules of study, for example those that cover areas such as law; social work methods; values and ethics; and the individual and society. The units/modules that you study on your degree will vary from programme to programme but whatever their title and content they are all designed to meet the overall academic and professional requirements of the social work degree, at either undergraduate or postgraduate level. Information about undertaking a literature search is contained in Chapter 5, *Analysing Information*.

6.4 ANALYSING AND ORGANISING THE MATERIAL

6.4.1 Analysing material

You will need to refer to Chapter 5 for guidelines and advice on analysing material. The areas included in that chapter that will help you to construct an assignment are: identifying appropriate material, learning to critique the literature, developing an argument and synthesising your ideas.

6.4.2 Organising the material

Step 1

Having undertaken some initial reading the planning list made by a student looked like this (Figure 6.1).

The plan captures key issues and areas for discussion.

Areas I need to consider in the assignment

THEORY and MODELS

Assessment models (e.g. Procedural, Exchange, Narrative etc.
(see Coulshed and Orme; Parker and Bradley)

1. Hierarchy of Needs (Maslow)

2. Social versus medical model of disability (Oliver and Sapey)

3. Person-centred practice (Rogers)

4. Communication Skills (Kaprowski)

5. Values, ethics (BASW, Banks, IFSW)

6. Anti-oppressive practice

LEGISLATION

National Assistance Act 1948

1. NHS and Community Care Act 1990

2. Direct Payments Act 1996

3. Carers Act 1995

4. Delayed Discharge Act 2005

5. Mental Capacity Act

POLICY

Fairer Access to Care 2006

1. Continuing Healthcare guidance 2010

2. Performance indicators CSCI 2006

3. Valuing People 2000

FIGURE 6.1 An example of a planning list produced by a student.

Step 2

However, to move forward into critical evaluation (as directed by the title) we need to do more than simply organise and describe the knowledge areas that make up the title: we need to explore some other, less tangible issues, tensions, puzzles and surprises. Puzzles and surprises arise out of the development of curiosity about the subject area. These might include ethical dilemmas in relation to person-centred practice in a context of budget constraints, inequalities in service delivery; conflicting political agendas, or conflicting views of authors.

6.4.3 Identifying tensions, puzzles and surprises

- Social care assessments are carried out by a range of professionals not just social workers – what different perspectives and skills might there be, and why?
- Political ideologies informing the NHS & CC Act.
- Might there be competing demands and tensions between needs-led and service-led assessments?
- Where does choice fit into the picture?
- What impact do eligibility criteria have?
- Inequalities e.g. 'Postcode lottery' of services and assessments.
- What is the purpose of social work – to relieve individual distress, maintain the status quo or promote social justice?
- What might be the impact of culture, power and oppression?
- How can anti-oppressive practice be demonstrated?
- Challenges of inter-professional and inter-agency working.

Step 3

Now we have some ideas – the next task is to begin to organise the information gathered. An essay normally has a three-part structure, the introduction, main body and conclusion.

 TOP TIP   Lecturer's tip

Rather than starting at what will be the beginning of the finished assignment and writing an introduction, try starting with a draft of the main body. The introduction can be written afterwards, when the content and direction of the assignment is clearer. You may deviate from your detailed plan as you continue to undertake wider reading and reflect on the material you have read and your introduction needs to accurately reflect the content.

Starting in the 'middle', leaving the introduction and conclusion until later can be useful, as introductions are far easier to write when you know what you have written. The introduction can be used to provide an initial overview telling the reader what will be included, what arguments will be used and an indication of what the essay will conclude. Waiting until you have a clear direction will save time and aid coherence.

By organising the information into themes, we will now consider how to create a structure that drives your arguments forward in a way that fulfils the requirements in the title and makes sense for the reader.

Here are some strategies described by current and past social work students. You may have your own strategies that work well for you.

- I draw up a plan, print it, then take a pair of scissors and cut up my plan into pieces that can be moved around, added to and considered in an interactive way.
- I type the key themes into boxes and move them around on the screen and keep adding to them.
- I use mind-mapping software.
- I make a plan then categorise and colour code all the sections of my notes according to which topic they belong in and then I start typing.
- I do lots of reading, make notes, think about what I've read and then start typing – I can move it around on the screen if I need to.
- I draw up a grid of sources I have read (using author, date, title, and website url) and note the key information. This helps me keep track of my sources.

6.5 CREATING A PLAN

This is the plan used by a student who completed the assignment we are using to illustrate this process.

1. Introduction – including identifying the chosen service user group.
2. The wider purpose of needs-led assessment in light of recent community care perspectives.
3. What the NHS and CC Act 1990 was, what it set out to achieve and issues using it in practice.
4. What is an assessment – national guidelines, policy, theories and models and assessment issues.
5. Practitioner influence on assessment and outcomes.
6. Oppression/empowerment – the role of values.
7. Conclusion.

STOP AND THINK...

Which aspect carries the most weight and which the least? Are marks attached to each section? Are a percentage of the marks awarded for analysis, content and presentation? How will you accommodate this in your plan?

It is important to plan for success. Re-familiarise yourself with the marking criteria for the specific assignment and the generic criteria for the level of study. Information about assessment criteria is included in Chapter 2 and you may want at this stage to revisit that chapter.

Taking the 2000-word example essay, you might consider breaking it down in the following way, to help you avoid writing too much or too little.

1 Introduction, 100 words

2 The wider purpose of needs, led assessment in light of recent community care perspectives, 150 words

3 The NHS and CC Act 1990, what it set out to achieve and challenges arising from using it in practice, 300 words

4 Identifying in more detail the context of a specific service user group, 150 words

5 Undertaking an assessment – national guidelines, policy, theories and models and assessment issues, 300 words

6 Practitioner influence on assessment and outcomes and implications for practice, 450 words

7 Oppression or empowerment and implications for practice, 450 words

8 Conclusion, 100 words

The student who shared this example reported that they immediately feel more confident about constructing an assignment after this stage as they have identified the sections where there is greater debate and allocated more words to them. It also helped them to begin to see the shape and structure of the assignment. You may notice that this form of plan contains content words rather than action and process words. At each level of your degree these are likely to be different to match the academic skills required to be demonstrated at each level (as we saw in Chapter 2), demonstrating increased analysis as you progress through the levels of the programme. It is important that you ensure you have fulfilled this part of expectations in the assignment title. In this assignment the process words are *evaluate, identify* and *illustrate*.

6.6 DEVELOPING A CLEAR STRUCTURE AND STYLE

As with the overall essay, each paragraph needs to contain a clear structure in order to lead the reader through the material and arguments. Each paragraph will contain one main topic area and constructing your assignment becomes much simpler when you approach it in an organised way. Williams (1995: 45) suggests the following format for building a paragraph.

- Topic sentence – to identify the main idea in the paragraph
- Provide clarification of any complex terminology
- Provide your evidence for the standpoint you have taken
- Critique the evidence by looking for others' explanations that either support or contradict your stance
- Widen the debate to demonstrate your ability to link information
- Consider unusual links to evidence your ability to consider information creatively and independently
- Note the implications of your argument
- Offer its importance in relation to your opening sentence.

We will illustrate the building of paragraphs using an actual assignment.

6.6.1 Paragraph 1

Prior to the NHS and Community Care Act 1990, services for adults with a learning disability were significantly different. Individuals lived in long-stay hospitals and care in the community might be more easily identified with the principles of care and containment (Valuing People 2000, and assessments focussed on the needs of the organisation rather than the individual.

Historically, according to Campbell and Oliver (1996), people with learning deficiencies were viewed in derogatory and discriminatory ways. Terms such as moron, idiot and, simpleton were used in legislation and policy documents and fell into common usage, indicating the lack of value placed on diversity or people who appeared different. As late as the 1970s and 1980s, residential homes were in the main, large with limited access to the community. Access to housing, education, and employment was minimal, and the term 'mental deficiency' reflected societal attitudes, stereotypes and norms (Valuing People 2000). The transformation to 'needs-led assessments' was sea-change in social care influenced by The Griffiths Report (1998), the White Paper, Caring for People (DoH 1989) and the resultant NHS and Community Care Act in 1990 (Bornat et al. 1997).

Lecturer's commentary

You need to think about how the first paragraph can continue the road map for the reader. You can see that the first sentence sets the scene. Can you see how it moves from this topic to the next point, the NHS and Community Care Act, using a linking sentence, which simply links one topic to another to aid the flow and coherence of the writing.

6.6.2 Paragraph 2

By implementing this legislation in 1993 the government intended to promote choice, inclusion and control for individuals in the assessment process.① The Act stated that 'case workers' not necessarily social workers would assess need and manage care planning. Thus the Care Manager was born. In addition, the focus of new language such as the 'mixed economy of care' highlighted the pivotal change from a state-led to competitively managed services encouraging the growth of private and voluntary sector solutions. In effect, the government anticipated that by re-inventing the client as the consumer, increased competition would improve quality and drive down costs (Means et al. 1998).② The legislation highlighted the importance of assessment to sensitively establish need whilst promoting inter-agency working and service user partnership. Consequently, some might argue the NHS and Community Care Act 1990 transformed policy and subsequently practice in assessment, quality control and costs. Assessment in particular became a pivotal aspect within care management processes. For instance, section 47 advised Local Authorities of their duty to undertake assessment of need, in relation to community care services, 'where an individual appears vulnerable'. However, this duty did not extend to discretionary services and as Braye and Preston-Shoot (1997) point out, case law accepted financial constraints as acceptable factors to take into account when providing services.③ This emerging picture appears to counter the 'transformational' arguments. Local Authorities could refuse provision if they were cash-strapped, and additionally, the act omitted to provide a definition of need, further enabling LAs to move from needs-led to crisis-reactive services. These conflicting tensions of needs versus resources continue to influence community care practice with practitioners required to balance individual need against scarce resources.④

Lecturer's commentary

We can re-examine this second paragraph using the numbered points in the paragraph to look at how the student has attempted to build an argument or debate and move forward.

① Here the main paragraph topic is placed at the forefront.

② In this section evidence from wider reading is provided from the standpoint being taken.

③ The student goes on to comment on the evidence by looking for literature that either supports or contradicts the stance. This widens the debate and demonstrates the ability to link information.

④ This identifies the implications for practice in the argument and links to the next paragraph.

6.6.3 Paragraph 3

The current philosophy of needs-led assessments for adults with learning disability remains a prerequisite of the NHS and Community Care Act 1990. However, whilst this remains the primary directive for assessment, there are tensions between its central aims of reducing expenditure and creating needs-led services (Means et al. 1998). Consequently, current constraints and practice dilemmas can lead to a disempowering services for adults with a learning disability (Means et al. 1998).

Lecturer's commentary

This is brief and to the point, informing the reader of a change in direction. In this case, the focus moves from past ideals to the present practice reality. The paragraph draws on the author's practice experience; let's consider this further.

The use of 'I'

Unless you are required to write a reflective account using the term 'I', the use of 'the first person' needs to be carefully considered to ensure you remain objective (see Chapter 3). You can see above where the student used the phrase 'in my experience'. On each occasion you move from an objective view to a subjective view it needs to be with good reason. In the paragraph example, the writer of the assignment has practice experience in this field and uses this to widen the debate. Each assignment should come with clear guidelines on the use of 'I', and in doubt always check with the lecturer responsible for the assignment.

6.6.4 Paragraph 4

Assessment of need is fundamental to care management and starts at the point of referral. Any individual, who appears in need, is offered an assessment to identify and measure the presenting need. The Department of Health guidelines (1990, cited Milner and O'Byrne 2002) instruct that assessments are 'simple, speedy and informal'. However, Gates (1999) suggests that gathering information to inform a full assessment for learning disabled adults is a formal and lengthy process. In addition the needs and views of a carer also have to be considered and may require their own assessment, a statutory duty, under The Carers (Recognition and Services) Act 1995. Whilst an assessment acknowledges the carers' need, in my experience services for carers are at best patchy, and at worst non-existent.

A fundamental pressurising factor in terms of assessment procedure currently is the Performance Assessment Framework Indicators (CSCI 2006 Standard D55). These government statistics indicate when an authority is not meeting its targets. Consequently the LA finds its funding adversely impacted upon, and it therefore becomes less and less able to provide timely, effective services. In my experience within learning disability services, practitioners face dilemmas around either meeting targets or compiling an assessment that is equitable and fair.

Lecturer's commentary

You can see how the opening sentence attempts to refer back to the title. The writer then attempts some *for and against* argument. They introduce carers, but this might be seen as a deviation from the assignment title and uses valuable words, although it demonstrates awareness of wider practice implications. Consider the 'for and against' section. Does this demonstrate evaluation, or is it descriptive? The latter part of the paragraph starts to engage critically with the issues. However, it stops. The marker's feedback said 'it would have been good to have seen how you could have expanded on this point'.

Where do you think it could be improved, and what are the strengths?

6.6.5 Paragraph 5

The tensions that impact upon assessment can be evident in the individual worker's approach to information gathering and analysis (Smale et al. 1993, cited Milner and O'Byrne1998). To meet performance targets, practitioners could feel pressurised into using a procedural model of assessment. Nonetheless despite time constraints, practitioners endeavour to continue a questioning approach in order to acknowledge and mitigate issues of power and structural oppression (Walker and Beckett 2005). Therefore, it remains crucial to consider and advocate methods of assessment that focus on best practice and empowerment, despite time and organisational constraints. One such assessment model (Fook 2002; p12) is the exchange model of assessment. By identifying the client as the expert in defining their problems, it highlights the practitioner skills of partnership working in order to enable the client to tell their story. Further, Smale et al. (1993, cited Milner and O'Byrne1998) cites this model as person-centred and potentially empowering. Moreover, they argue it enhances national directives including the NHS and Community Act 1990, and good practice guidance such as the Valuing People (2000) White Paper. Concurring, Parker and Bradley (2005) suggest adopting this approach to enable practitioners to focus on individual need rather than become overwhelmed by agency requirements. There appears a strong argument that this model assists workers to remain congruent with social work values as it places the person at the heart of the assessment. From my experience in a statutory learning disability team, practitioners are indeed empowered by the use of this model. It enables a person-centred approach that then informs our interpretation of local policy and national guidance. At present, our assessments explore individual strengths before needs, and obtain information from the individual and others they see as important in their life. This approach also promotes task-centred practice, enabling meaningful individual goal setting to be established through the assessment process. It would appear that by respecting people's legitimate claim to independence, choice, rights and inclusion (Valuing People 2000), this form of community care assessment approach enhances people's opportunity to live a fair and equitable life. Of course there are constraints, tensions and conflict to consider both at an individual and societal perspective. However, the growth of advocacy aims to address and minimise conflicts, particularly in circumstances where the service user's rights are in conflict with agency constraints.

Introducing debates enhances the discussion and moves from description to analysis. Look at the paragraph again and identify the words you believe help to direct the debate.

Lecturer's commentary

What words did you jot down?

Your list might have included some of the following phrases:

- To show place – above, below, here, there, etc.
- To show time – after, before, currently, during, earlier, later, etc.

- To give an example – for example, for instance, etc.
- To show addition – additionally, also, and, furthermore, moreover, equally important, etc.
- To show similarity – also, likewise, in the same way, similarly, etc.
- To show an exception – but, however, nevertheless, on the other hand, on the contrary, yet, etc.
- To show a sequence – first, second, third, next, then, etc.
- To emphasise – indeed, in fact, of course, etc.
- To show cause and effect – accordingly, consequently, therefore, thus, etc.
- To conclude or repeat – finally, in conclusion, on the whole, in the end, etc.

(Gocsik 2005)

6.6.6 Paragraph 6

Oppression or empowerment

The success of community care assessment is influenced by practitioners' advocacy skills. This in turn is often dependent on an individual practitioner's skills, values and beliefs. Demonstrating values of respect, confidentiality and honesty enhances assessment approaches but these can be affected by factors such as lack of knowledge, inexperience or differing levels of professional integrity. Social work values are the cornerstone of good practice, but one key aspect of the NHS and Community Care Act 1990 was the introduction of Care Managers. This has led to a variety of associated professionals, teachers, nurses or occupational therapists bringing their diverse professional skills to the community care assessment process. When our values and skills are congruent, this diversity enhances the experience of clients. However, distinct approaches towards assessment require further consideration. One good example is the Fair Access to Care Services policy (FACS 2006) which sets out four graduating levels of needs and resulting service response. Locally thresholds move in response of funding constraints. This resource-orientated shift means accurate and meaningful assessment becomes ever more critical to ensure individuals receive a true assessment of their need. Consequently, it is important to note how individual assessors may interpret need dependent on their professional training and core values. For example the NMC Code of Conduct (S8 2004) highlights the importance of 'minimising risk to patients and clients', whilst in contrast, the GSCC (2002: 4.1) focuses on, 'recognising that clients have the right to take risks'. Whilst these principles of practice overlap, they also highlight how training can promote either an enabling or oppressing style of practice. Hornby and Atkins (2000) concur, citing their theory of formation of professional identity. They evidence how early practitioner experiences, attitudes and stereotypes inform and shape future practice. Further, the social and medical models of disability influence training that shape professional intervention. This is not to suggest that all nurses view people in terms of their illness or disability, nor that all social workers understand and act upon inequality and discrimination, rather to highlight that training subconsciously informs assessment perspectives. In light of this, it becomes evermore crucial that community care assessment approaches are used in conjunction with social work core values. One piece of legislation charged with improving this area of inequality was the Direct Payments Act 1996. Disability rights organisations such as People First campaigned for the introduction of genuine independence, choice and control within community care. The Act aimed to provide people with cash payments to empower and enable self-organisation of services. This was commonly viewed (Oliver and Sapey 1999, cited Glasby et al. 2002) as the most fundamental reorganisation of welfare for half a century. However, in practice this remains difficult to achieve again due in part to resource constraints and institutionalised systems and procedures. Nevertheless, when used successfully it is possible to see Maslow's hierarchy of needs evident through individual progression and achievement of steps towards self-actualisation.

Lecturer's commentary

The paragraph has covered a lot of ground. It would be strengthened by references to the literature on inter-agency and inter-professional working (for example, see Quinney and Hafford-Letchfield 2012 or Pollard et al. 2010). A reference for the information about People First is needed.

Some analysis of the impact of direct payments and the personalisation agenda would be helpful – has it improved quality of life and led to choice and independence?

The mention of Maslow at the end needs development. Whilst it is useful to draw on material from psychology and sociology this point needs a reference and it is also important to note that the notion of self-actualisation is contested.

There is good use of signposting, analysis and summarisation.

6.6.7 Writing the conclusion

One approach is to look backwards. Consider what you have written and consider how the question has been answered. Some students approach the conclusion as a statement or summary of the content by indicating how the title has been answered. An alternative approach involves focussing on the new insights you have developed from the synthesis of ideas and highlighting new approaches to the material, and in doing so it looks forward rather than backwards.

> This essay has explored a range of key principles affecting the use of a community care assessment approach with adults with a learning disability. It has examined legislation and government directives that whilst intending to promote social justice can through implementation actually add to the oppression of socially disadvantaged groups. This may be caused in some part, through the structures and objectives of local authorities which unintentionally conflict with the principles of choice, control and independence enshrined in Valuing People (2000). This can become even more contentious when assessment of need is subject to local definition and resource issues. Additionally the differing values held by practitioners further impact upon outcomes for adults with learning disabilities. It would seem that both challenges and opportunities have been created through recent legislation and guidance. In conclusion, the essay demonstrates the importance of practitioners' ability to navigate their way through competing tensions to ensure assessments are person-centred and needs led. Assessments remain central to the care management process and it is the practitioner skills, knowledge and experience which enables a genuinely empowering outcome.

Lecturer's commentary

Consider these suggestions by Gocsik (2005)

- Review the background information with which you began, and illustrate how your argument has shed new light on that information.
- Return to the key terms and point out how your essay has added some new dimension to their meanings.
- Use a quotation that summarises or reflects your main idea.
- Acknowledge your opponent's point of view – if only to emphasise that you've provided an alternative position.

- Remember: language is especially important to a conclusion. Your goal in your final sentences is to leave your ideas resounding in your reader's mind. Give them something to think about. Make your language ring.

You can also revisit the checklists for critical thinking and writing, and reflection and reflective writing in Chapters 3 and 4.

6.6.8 Writing the introduction

Having written the main body of the assignment we now need to set the scene, establish the wider picture and focus, grab the reader's attention and signpost them to the main body. Writing the introduction should not be done in a hurry. This is your chance to capture interest, to make the reader want to read on as well as being required to read on in order to mark your work and provide feedback). Gimenez (2007) considers the written style that readers of the English language will find most persuasive. Interestingly, he reports that readers prefer to hear a topic overview before developing a focus for the assignment. Quite simply, Gimenez (2007: 5) advises that you should provide your *'background information'* before your *'focus'*. Next, explain why you are approaching the assignment in a particular way – your *'rationale'*. Lastly, *'signpost'* your reader through the journey of your argument – both the debate you will have (informative) and the process you have taken (discussion/analysis/evaluation).

Let's look at the introduction in the example essay.

> The growing importance of evidence-based practice in social care has implications for all aspects of service provision including needs-led assessments, and demonstrates where practice either oppresses or empowers.
>
> This essay examines the nature and purpose of community care assessments for adults with a learning disability, focussing on factors influencing practitioner approaches. To achieve this the essay will firstly outline recent historical contexts, examine the broader aims of legislation and consider practice dilemmas and their impact on individuals and their assessment. The essay will consider some fundamental issues affecting assessments. These will include examining at a broader level how individual differences, assessment models and the reality of balancing rights against scarce resources influence assessment. Finally, at a micro level, the essay moves on to consider other influences such as values, oppression and opportunity, before weighing up the impact of competing principles and tensions on needs-led assessments.
>
> For the purposes of this work, assessment is defined as 'to judge the worth or importance of' (Collins 1995: 50) and need, 'to require or be in want of' (Collins 1995: 637).
>
> The essay acknowledges the impact of partner agencies and other professionals that carry out assessments such as those from Health or Occupational Therapy services, but word constraints limit the discussion to areas that would normally form part of a community care assessment. Throughout, issues of diversity will be highlighted and the theories and values that explain and challenge behaviour will be identified. It should be noted that the viewpoints and beliefs held by the writer are a result of personal life experiences, ideology and worldview; they are Euro-centric and may differ from the readers' own perspectives.

Lecturer's commentary

Has this introduction achieved the following?

- Interpreted the approach to the question being taken
- Highlighted the debates and major topic areas

- Defined key terms
- Established the writer's position in relation to the assignment title
- Signposted accurately

TOP TIP

Try to avoid referring to the limitations of the word count – this takes up valuable words in itself. It is better to clearly and confidently state the scope of the assignment.

6.7 REVIEWING, PROOFREADING AND EDITING

Having written your assignment you might feel relieved but the work is not over yet! There are some more steps before you can submit the assignment. Set aside plenty of time for this stage.

6.7.1 Step 1: Reviewing the overall content

One excellent piece of advice Williams (1995) offers is to consider what you have written in light of what you have been trying to achieve. Does your assignment demonstrate your knowledge and understanding for the reader?

Could you examine the material in a different way, perhaps consider it from the perspective of another? Critically reflecting on your work, as Williams (1995) suggests from an alternative view-point, can develop your assignment in a way which demonstrates your personal take on an issue or subject area. Avoid simplistic answers or conclusions; social work is complex and contested and your work should reflect this.

Check that you have avoided digressing from the question by ensuring that you have answered the question and addressed the ILOs. Review your structure and consider the flow of your argument. Can you see connections within and between paragraphs –with topics flowing into the next? Does the main body follow the plan you have set out in the introduction; does the conclusion explain how you answered the question?

6.7.2 Step 2: Looking at the detail by proofreading

Having reviewed what you have produced you now have the opportunity to look in detail at the assignment and proofread and edit your assignment in order to strengthen it.

Allow plenty of time for proofreading. By proofreading on the screen you can note any queries your word processing programme has identified, such as spelling, punctuation and grammar. Ensure you have set your spellchecker to British and not American English, and take care with the choices the spellchecker offers. If in doubt check the meaning and correct spelling in a dictionary.

Poor spelling, punctuation and grammar detracts from an otherwise sound assignment, and students bring very different experiences of the rules of written English to assignment writing. Matt, despite his academic anxieties, had absorbed the rules of punctuation during secondary education whereas Sarah's academic experience was significant as an adult learner but limited at secondary school level and consequently many basic writing skills, including spelling rules and the use of punctuation, had to be learnt as an adult. If this is you, please don't worry. There are resources available to check and learn English grammar, such as those recommended at the end of the chapter, and you will become more aware of the rules of writing as you begin to read widely. Like any other aspects of writing, punctuation is a series of rules.

After proofreading on a computer screen you might find it useful to print off your work and read it aloud. Reading aloud slows down the pace of reading and can help you identify errors that you have missed.

6.7.3 Step 3: Editing

Look for and remove

- Information that is irrelevant to the title and ILOs
- Repeat information

Look for and insert

- Missing references (ensure the references in the text match those in the reference list)
- Missing coverage of key arguments.

Have you written too many words?
Edit the assignment by removing unnecessary words. For example

They are in fact	replace with	in fact
Very relevant	replace with	relevant
Few in number	replace with	few

Edit the assignment by removing unnecessary phrases. For example

In view of the fact that	replace with	because
Are of the same opinion	replace with	agree
In spite of the fact that	replace with	although

Check the length of your sentences. If a sentence is more than 30 words long consider how you might shorten it by removing unnecessary words or phrases. Short sentences can be used to provide impact.

You might want to ask a friend or 'study buddy' to read it through and point out any spelling and grammar errors, and to comment on the clarity of the argument and logical structure of the material.

6.7.4 Step 4: Check the references

Accurate referencing is essential. The reference list indicates the breadth and depth of the research and reading that underpins the assignment. It is important to clearly distinguish between your ideas and those in the sources you have read, and to acknowledge the authors whose work informs the assignment. Lecture notes are normally seen as triggers to further reading. Do check the conventions and requirements of the programme you are following to establish whether references to lecture notes is permitted.

Building your reference list as you develop your assignment ensures you don't miss any sources used. Each time you refer to a source you must add it to the reference list, to ensure that the in-text references match the reference list.

It is essential that you follow the referencing guidelines provided by your programme or university about the format for setting out your references. Avoid simply copying the reference as it appears in the reference list of a book, journal article, or other source as they may be using a different format.

Anne, a social work lecturer, comments

When I mark assignments I start with the reference list. This might seem rather 'back to front', but a reference list is a very good indicator of the depth and breadth of reading that has been undertaken and literature that will be drawn on to underpin the arguments presented.

Always take care with constructing a reference list and ensure all the references in the text are included in and accurately match the reference list, and that it is constructed by following the guide you have been provided with. Not all universities use exactly the same format, and the format used in the textbooks and peer-reviewed journal articles you have read will not necessarily be in the same style that you are expected to use.

6.7.5 Step 5: Make a final check of the title and ILOs

Check that you have done what was required, that you have fully answered the question. This can be done in a very practical way.

Take the title again

> Using a Community Care assessment approach outline and evaluate the key principles underpinning the assessment process outlined in government legislation and national policy documents. Identify any social work theories and values that might influence your assessment. Illustrate your answer with reference to one particular service user group.

Transfer this into a checklist and make brief notes to yourself about the extent to which you have covered the key areas.

Have you outlined and evaluated the following?

Community Care assessment process

Underpinning key principles

Legislation and policy

Theories (which ones?)

Values (which ones?)

One service user group

CONCLUSION

By following the format identified in this chapter, you will be able to produce a credible essay that has a clear structure and flow.

Sarah's comment:

When I began to approach assignment writing in this organised way I gained higher marks, and left university with a first class degree. I often reflect back on my feelings of uncertainty when trying to write assignments. In fact I'm experiencing similar feelings when writing this book. There are others areas in life that do not come easily – cleaning and maths, for example – but this does not disturb me; in fact I often celebrate my disinterest and lack of skill in areas such as housework and there are other people at home who are understanding and more accomplished. When I'm writing, it seems important to me that I am excellent immediately. It's not realistic, but I take heart, and I hope you will too, in the knowledge that like learning any new skill I can improve if I only take the time to practice. I believe that good assignment writing for most people is not an innate skill and something that comes easily, but the result of perseverance and determination to develop and succeed, using feedback and support.

With practise, you too will begin to feel more comfortable with researching, planning, structuring and organising the material and this will lead to higher marks.

FURTHER READING

Healy, L. and Mulholland, J. 2002. *Writing skills for social workers*. London: Sage.

Trask, R.L. 2004. *Penguin guide to punctuation*. London: Penguin.

Truss, L. 2005. *Eats, shoots and leaves: the zero tolerance approach to punctuation*. London: Profile Books.

REFERENCES

Adams, R., Dominelli, L. and Payne, M. (Eds). 2002. *Themes, issues and critical debates.* 2nd ed. Basingstoke: Palgrave.

Adams, R., Dominelli, L. and Payne, M. (Eds). 2005. *Social work futures; crossing boundaries, transforming practice.* Basingstoke: Palgrave.

Adams, R., Dominelli, L. and Payne, M. (Eds). 2009. *Critical practice in social work.* Basingstoke: Palgrave.

Argyris, C. 1999. *On organizational learning.* Oxford: Blackwell.

Ash, S., Clayton, P. and Moses, M. 2006. Schematic overview of the DEAL model for critical reflection. *Teaching and learning through critical reflection: an instructor's guide.* Sterling, VA: Stylus Publishing.

ASKe. undated a. *Using generic feedback effectively.* Oxford Brookes University. Available from www.business.brookes.ac.uk/aske.html

ASKe. undated b. *Assessment. Doing better.* Oxford Brookes University. Available from www.business.brookes.ac.uk/aske.html

Audit Commission. 2002. *Recruitment and retention: a public service workforce for the 20th century.* London: Audit Commission.

Banks, S. 2012. *Values and ethics in social work.* 4th ed. Basingstoke: Palgrave Macmillan.

Barnett, R. 1997. *Higher education: a critical business.* Buckingham: SRHE/Open University Press.

Baxter Magolda, M.B. 1992. *Knowing and reasoning in college: gender related patterns in students' intellectual development.* San Francisco: Jossey-Bass.

Bellinger, A. 2010.Talking about (re)generation: practice leaning as a site for renewal of social work. *British Journal of Social Work* 40, 2450–66.

Bogo, M., Regehr, C., Katz, E., Logie, C. and Mylopoulos, M. 2011. Developing a tool for assessing students' reflections on their practice. *Social Work Education* 30(2), 186–94.

Boud, D. 1993. Experience as the base for learning. *Studies in Continuing Education* 12(1), 33–44.

British Association of Social Workers (BASW). 2012. *The code of ethics for social work; statement of principles.* Birmingham: BASW

Brown, K. and Rutter, L. 2006. *Critical thinking for social work.* Exeter: Learning Matters.

Brown, K. and Rutter, L. 2008. *Critical thinking for social work.* 2nd Ed. Exeter: Learning Matters.

Bye, L., Smith, S. and Monaghan Rallis, H. 2009. Reflection using an online discussion forum: impact on student learning and satisfaction. *Social Work Education* 28(8), 841–55.

Calvin Thomas, G. and Howe, K. 2011. Supporting black and minority ethnic students in practice learning. *The Journal of Practice Teaching and Learning* 10(3), 41–58.

Centre for Human Services Technology. 2005. *Researchmindedness.* Southampton: University of Southampton. Available from www.resmind.swap.ac.uk

Christie, A. (Ed). 2001. *Men in social work.* Abingdon: Routledge.

College of Social Work. 2012 a. *The professional capability framework for social work.* London: College of Social Work. Available from: www.collegeofsocialwork.org/pcf.aspx

College of Social Work. 2012 b. *Developing your social work practice using the PCF.* London: College of Social Work. Available from: www.collegeofsocialwork.org/uploadedFiles/TheCollege/Media_centre/PCF21IntegratedCriticalReflectivePractice(1).pdf.

Collins, S., Coffey, M. and Morris, L. 2010. Social work students: stress, support and wellbeing. *The British Journal of Social Work* 40(3), 963–82.

Cooper, A., Lymbery, M., Ruch, G. and Wilson, K. 2008. *Social work; an introduction to contemporary practice.* Harlow: Pearson Education.

Cottrell, S. 2005. *Critical thinking skills.* Basingstoke: PalgraveMacmillan.

Cottrell, S. 2011. *Critical thinking skills.* 2nd ed. London: Palgrave.

Coyle, M., and Peck, J., 2005. *Write it Right: A Handbook for Students.* Palgrave Macmillan: Hampshire.

Cree, V. 2000. The challenge of assessment. In: *Transfer of learning in professional and vocational education.* Cree, V. and McCauley, C. (Eds). Routledge: London.

Cree, V. (Ed). 2003. *Becoming a social worker.* Abingdon: Routledge.

Cree, V. and Davis, A. (Eds). 2007. *Voices from the inside.* Abingdon: Routledge.

Cree, V. with Doyle, F., Lough, L., Mecandante, I., Peat, L. and Robertson, G. 2006. Innovation in social work students' assessment. *Social Work Education* 25(2), 189–91.

Dempsey, M., Halton, C. and Murphy, M. 2001. Reflective learning in social work education: scaffolding the process. *Social Work Education* 20(6), 631–41.

Department of Health. 2002. *Requirements for social work training.* London: DoH.

Dewey, J. 1933. *How we think.* Lexington, MA: D.C. Heath.

Doel, M. and Shardlow, S. 1995. *Modern social work practice: teaching and learning in practice settings.* Aldershot: Ashgate.

Doel, M. and Shardlow, S. 1996. *Social work in a changing world: an international perspective on practice learning.* Aldershot: Ashgate.

Elder, L. and Paul, R. 2006. *The miniature guide to critical thinking concepts and tools.* The foundation for critical thinking. Available from www.criticalthinking.org/files/Concepts_Tools.pdf.

Fenge, L.A., Hughes, M., Howe, K. and Thomas, G. 2012. *Practice learning portfolios in social work: a handbook.* Maidenhead: Open University Press.

Fisher, M. and Marsh, P. 2005. *Developing the evidence base for social work and social care practice.* London: SCIE.

Fook, J. 2002. *Social work; a critical approach to practice.* London: Sage.

Fook, J. 2012. *Social work; a critical approach to practice.* 2nd ed. London: Sage.

Fook, J. and Askeland, G. 2007. Challenges of critical reflection; 'nothing ventured, nothing gained'. *Social Work Education* 26(5), 520–33.

General Social Care Council. 2010. *Raising standards. Social work education in England 2008–09.* London: General Social Care Council.

Gibbs, G. 1988. *Learning by doing: a guide to teaching and learning methods.* Oxford: Further Education Unit, Oxford Polytechnic.

Gimenez, J. 2007. *Writing for nursing and midwifery students.* Basingstoke: Palgrave. Macmillan

Gocsik, K., 2005. Materials for students. Dartmouth writing program. www.dartmouth.edu/~writing/materials/student/ac_paper/write.shtml

Golding, C. 2011. Educating for critical thinking: thought-encouraging questions in a community of enquiry. *Higher Education Research and Development* 30(3), 357–70.

Greasley P and Cassidy A 2009. When it comes round to marking assignments: how to impress and how to 'distress' lecturers. *Assessment and Evaluation in Higher Education.* 35 (2), 173–189.

Green Lister, P. 2012. *Integrating social work theory and practice.* London: Routledge.

Green Lister, P. and Crisp, B. 2007. Critical incident analyses: a practice learning tool for students and practitioners. *Practice* 19(1), 47–60.

Green Lister, P., Dutton, K. and Crisp, B.R. 2005. Assessment practices in Scottish social work education: a practice audit of Scottish universities providing qualifying social work. *Social Work Education* 24(6), 693–711.

Hart, C. 1998. *Doing a literature review.* London: Sage.

Healy, K. 2005. *Social work theories in context; creating frameworks for practice.* Basingstoke: Palgrave.

Heron, G. 2006. Critical thinking in social care and social work: searching student assignments for the evidence. *Social Work Education* 25(3), 209–24.

Holstrom, C. and Taylor, I. 2008. Researching admissions: what can we learn about selection of applicants from findings about students in difficulty on a social work programme. *Social Work Education* 27(8), 819–36.

Hudson, J. 2010. *Programme-level assessment. A review of selected material.* University of Bradford. Available from www.pass.brad.ac.uk

Humphries, B. 2008. *Social work research for social justice.* Basingstoke: Palgrave Macmillan.

Hussein, S., Moriarty, J. and Manthorpe, J. 2009. *Variations in the progression of social work students in England.* Social Care Workforce Research Unit. London: Kings College London/GSCC.

Hutchings, M., Quinney, A., Galvin, K. and Clarke, V. 2012. The yin/yang of innovative technology enhanced assessment for promoting student learning. In *Proceedings of the 11th European Conference on Elearning.* Groningen, Netherlands.

IASSW/IFSW.2004. Ethics in social work: statement of principles. Available from http://ifsw.org/policies/statement-of-ethical-principles/

International Association of Schools of Social Work and International Federation of Social Workers. 2000. *Definition of social work.* IASSW/IFSW. Available from http://ifsw.org/policies/definition-of-social-work

Kolb, D.A. 1984. *Experiential learning: experience as the source of learning and development.* Englewood Cliffs, NJ: Prentice Hall.

Kolb, D.A. 1993. *Learning styles inventory-IIa: self scoring inventory and interpretation booklet.* Boston: McBer & Company.

Laming, Lord. 2009. *The protection of children in England: A progress report.* London: TSO.

Lay, K. and McGuire, L. 2010. Building a lens for critical reflection and reflexivity in social work education. *Social Work Education* 29(5), 539–50.

Liverpool John Moores University. 2008. *Effective practice in assessment.* 3rd ed. Liverpool: Liverpool John Moores University Learning and Teaching Development Unit.

Martyn, H. 2006. *Developing reflective practice. Making sense of social work in a world of change.* Bristol: The Policy Press.

McCann, L. and Saunders, S. Undated. *Exploring student perceptions of assessment feedback.* Southampton: The Higher Education Academy Subject Centre for Social Policy and Social Work (SWAP).

Moon, J. 1999. *Reflection in learning and professional development: theory and practice.* London: Kogan Page.

Moon, J. 2004. *A handbook of reflective and experiential learning. Theory and practice.* London: Routledge.

Moon, J. 2005. *We seek it here … a new perspective on the elusive activity of critical thinking: a theoretical and practical approach.* Bristol: Escalate Higher Education Academy.

Moriarty, J. and Murray, L. 2007. Who wants to be a social worker? Using routine published data to identify trends in the numbers of people applying for and completing social work programmes in England. *British Journal of Social Work* 37, 715–33.

Parrott, L. 2006. *Values and ethics in social work practice.* Exeter: Learning Matters.

Pawson, R., Boaz, A., Grayson, L., Long, A. and Barnes, C. 2003. *Types and quality of knowledge in social care.* Knowledge review 3. London: Social Care Institute for Excellence.

Payne, M. 2005. *Modern social work theory.* 2nd ed. Basingstoke: Palgrave.

Payne, M. 2006. *What is professional social work?* Bristol: BASW/Policy Press.

Perry, R. and Cree, V. 2003. The changing gender profile of applicants to qualifying social work training in the UK. *Social Work Education* 22(4), 375–83.

Pollard K.C., Thomas J. and Miers M. (Eds). 2010 *Understanding interprofessional. working in health and social care*. Basingstoke: Palgrave Macmillan.

Preston-Shoot, M. 1996. Whither social work? Social work, social policy and law at an interface: confronting the challenges and realising the potential in work with people needing care or services. *The Liverpool Law Review* XVIII(1), 19–39.

Pulman, A., Galvin, G., Hutchings, M., Todres, L., Quinney, A., Ellis-Hill, C. and Atkins, P. 2012. Empathy and dignity through technology: using lifeworld-led multimedia to enhance learning about the head, hand and heart. *Electronic Journal of Elearning* 10(3), 349–59.

Quality Assurance Agency. 2008. *Subject benchmark statement: social work*. Gloucester: QAA.

Quinney, A. 2005. 'Placements online': student experiences of a website to support learning in practice settings. *Social Work Education* 24(4), 439–50.

Quinney, A. 2008. Introducing formative assessment tool. *Focus* (Winter), 8–9. Southampton: The Higher Education Academy Subject Centre for Social Policy and Social Work (SWAP). Available from: www.swap.ac.uk/docs/newsletters/infocus01_online.pdf

Quinney, A. and Hafford-Letchfield, P. 2012. *Interprofessional social work: effective collaborative approaches*. London: Sage.

Quinney, A. and Parker, J. 2010. Developing self-efficacy in research skills: becoming research-minded. In: *The outcomes of social work education; developing evaluation methods*. Monograph 2. Southampton: The Higher Education Academy Subject Centre for Social Policy and Social Work.

Quinney, A., Hutchings, M. and Pulman, A. 2012. Faciltiating critical reflection and the empathic imagination using arts and humanities material: exploring knowledge for the head, hand and heart. Paper given at the Joint Social Work Education and Research Conference (JSWEC) Manchester.

Quinney, A., Thomas, J. and Whittington, C. 2009. *Interprofessional and interagency collaboration*. London: Social Care Institute for Excellence. Available from www.scie.org.uk/publications/elearning/ipiac/index.asp

Redman, P. and Maples, W. 2011. *Good essay writing in the social sciences*. London: Sage.

Redman, P. 2001. *Good Essay Writing. A Social Sciences Guide*. The Open University: Milton Keynes.

Roberts, S. 2011. Traditional practice for non-traditional students? Examining the role of pedagogy in higher education retention. *Journal of Further and Higher Education* 35(2), 183–99.

Rose, J., 2007. *The Mature Student's Guide to Writing*. 2nd ed. Palgrave Macmillan: Hampshire.

Rust, C. 2007. Towards a scholarship of assessment. *Assessment & Evaluation in Higher Education* 32(2), 126–31.

Rutter, L. and Williams, S. 2007. *Enabling and assessing work-based learning for social work. Supporting the development of professional practice*. Birmingham: Learn to Care.

Schon, D. 1991. *Educating the reflective practitioner: towards a new design for teaching and learning in the professions*. Oxford: Jossey-Bass.

Schon, D.A.1983. *The reflective practitioner; how professionals think in action*. New York: Basic Books.

Schon, D. 1996. *The reflective practitioner: how professionals think in action*. Aldershot: Arena.

Shardlow, S. 2002. Values, ethics and social work. In: Adams, R., Dominelli, L. and Payne, M. (Eds). *Social work: themes, issues and critical debates*. Basingstoke: Palgrave.

Shaw, I.F. 1985. A closed profession? Recruitment to social work. *British Journal of Social Work* 15(3), 261–80.

Singh, G. 2001. To be or not to be competent, that is the question; putting the horse before the cart – developing assessment driven by learning rather than by regulation. Paper for the 3rd Annual Practice Learning and Teaching Conference, 23 November 2001, Nottingham.

SWAP. 2007. *The social work degree: preparing to succeed.* SWAP Guide 3. Southampton: SWAP.

SWAP. 2008. *What makes a good lecturer? The student perspective.* SWAP Guide 4b. Southampton: The Higher Education Academy Subject Centre for Social Policy and Social Work (SWAP).

Taylor, C. and White, S. 2006. Knowledge and reasoning in social work: educating for humane judgement. *British Journal of Social Work* 36(6), 937–54.

The Telegraph. 2012. Available from www.telegraph.co.uk/news/politics/9049505/Days-lost-to-strikes-hit-20-year-high.html.

Thomas, J., Quinney, A. and Whittington, C. 2009. *Building relationships, establishing trust and working with others.* London: Social Care Institute for Excellence.

Thomson, N. 2000. *Understanding social work: preparing for practice.* Basingstoke: Palgrave.

Trevithick, P. 2012. *Social work skills and knowledge; a practice handbook.* London: McGraw Hill.

UNISON, 2012. Available from www.unison.org.uk/paymatters/whystrike.asp.

Walter, I., Nutley, S., Percy-Smith, J., McNeish, D. and Frost, S. 2004. *Improving the use of research in social care practice.* SCIE Knowledge review 07. London: SCIE.

Warren, J. 2007. *Service user and carer participation in social work.* Exeter: Learning Matters.

Wayne, J., Bogo, M. and Raskin, M. 2010. Field education as the signature pedagogy of social work education: congruence and disparity. *Journal of Social Work Education* 46(3), 327–39.

Whittington, C., Thomas, J. and Quinney, A. 2009. *Professional identity and collaboration.* London: Social Care Institute for Excellence.

Williams, K., 1995. *Writing essays: developing writing.* The Oxford Centre for Staff Development: Oxford.

Wilson, K., Ruch, G., Lymbery, M. and Cooper, A. with Becker, S., Bell, M., Brammer, A., Clawson, R., Littlechild, B., Paylor, I. and Smith, R. 2011. *Social work. An introduction to contemporary practice.* 2nd ed. London: Pearson.

Wolf, K. 2010. Bridging the distance: the use of blogs as reflective learning tools for placement students. *Higher Education Research and Development* 29(5), 589–602.

Worsley, A., Stanley, N., O'Hare, P., Keeler, A., Cooper, L. and Hollowell, C. 2009. Great expectations; the growing divide between students and social work educators. *Social Work Education* 28(8), 828–40.

APPENDIX 1
THE COLLEGE OF SOCIAL WORK DOMAINS WITHIN THE PCF

The Professional Capabilities Framework has nine domains (or areas) within it. For each one, there is a main statement and an elaboration. Then at each level within the PCF, detailed capabilities have been developed explaining how social workers should expect to evidence that area in practice.

The nine capabilities should be seen as interdependent, not separate. As they interact in professional practice, so there are overlaps between the capabilities within the domains, and many issues will be relevant to more than one domain. Understanding of what a social worker does will only be complete by taking into account all nine capabilities.

Professionals and their practice will be assessed 'holistically', by which we mean that throughout their careers, social work students and practitioners need to demonstrate integration of all aspects of learning, and provide a sufficiency of evidence across all nine domains.

1. PROFESSIONALISM – Identify and behave as a professional social worker, committed to professional development

Social workers are members of an internationally recognised profession, a title protected in UK law. Social workers demonstrate professional commitment by taking responsibility for their conduct, practice and learning, with support through supervision. As representatives of the social work profession they safeguard its reputation and are accountable to the professional regulator.

2. VALUES AND ETHICS – Apply social work ethical principles and values to guide professional practice

Social workers have an obligation to conduct themselves ethically and to engage in ethical decision making, including through partnership with people who use their services. Social workers are knowledgeable about the value base of their profession, its ethical standards and relevant law.

3. DIVERSITY – Recognise diversity and apply anti-discriminatory and anti-oppressive principles in practice

Social workers understand that diversity characterises and shapes human experience and is critical to the formation of identity. Diversity is multi-dimensional and includes race, disability, class, economic status, age, sexuality, gender and transgender, faith and belief. Social workers appreciate that, as a consequence of difference, a person's life experience may include oppression, marginalisation and alienation as well as privilege, power and acclaim, and are able to challenge appropriately.

4. RIGHTS, JUSTICE AND ECONOMIC WELLBEING – Advance human rights and promote social justice and economic wellbeing

Social workers recognise the fundamental principles of human rights and equality, and that these are protected in national and international law, conventions and policies. They ensure these principles underpin their practice. Social workers understand the importance of using and contributing to case law and applying these rights in their own practice. They understand the effects of oppression, discrimination and poverty.

5. KNOWLEDGE – Apply knowledge of social sciences, law and social work practice theory

Social workers understand psychological, social, cultural, spiritual and physical influences on people; human development throughout the life span and the legal framework for practice. They apply this knowledge in their work with individuals, families and communities. They know and use theories and methods of social work practice.

6. CRITICAL REFLECTION AND ANALYSIS – Apply critical reflection and analysis to inform and provide a rationale for professional decision making

Social workers are knowledgeable about and apply the principles of critical thinking and reasoned discernment. They identify, distinguish, evaluate and integrate multiple sources of knowledge and evidence. These include practice evidence, their own practice experience, service user and carer experience together with research-based, organisational, policy and legal knowledge. They use critical thinking augmented by creativity and curiosity.

7. INTERVENTION AND SKILLS – Use judgement and authority to intervene with individuals, families and communities to promote independence, provide support and prevent harm, neglect and abuse

Social workers engage with individuals, families, groups and communities, working alongside people to assess and intervene. They enable effective relationships and are effective communicators, using appropriate skills. Using their professional judgement, they employ a range of interventions: promoting independence, providing support and protection, taking preventative action and ensuring safety whilst balancing rights and risks. They understand and take account of differentials in power, and are able to use authority appropriately. They evaluate their own practice and the outcomes for those they work with.

8. CONTEXTS AND ORGANISATIONS – Engage with, inform, and adapt to changing contexts that shape practice. Operate effectively within own organisational frameworks and contribute to the development of services and organisations. Operate effectively within multi-agency and inter-professional settings

Social workers are informed about and pro-actively responsive to the challenges and opportunities that come with changing social contexts and constructs. They fulfil this responsibility in accordance with their professional values and ethics, both as individual professionals and as members of the organisation in which they work. They collaborate, inform and are informed by their work with others, inter-professionally and with communities.

9. PROFESSIONAL LEADERSHIP – Take responsibility for the professional learning and development of others through supervision, mentoring, assessing, research, teaching, leadership and management

The social work profession evolves through the contribution of its members in activities such as practice research, supervision, assessment of practice, teaching and management. An individual's contribution will gain influence when undertaken as part of a learning, practice-focussed organisation. Learning may be facilitated with a wide range of people including social work colleagues, service users and carers, volunteers, foster carers and other professionals.

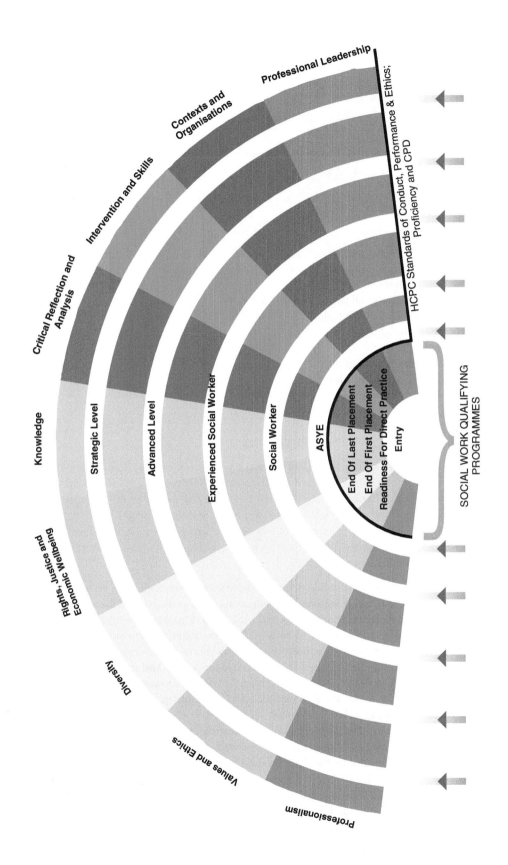

Professional Leadership

Contexts and Organisations

Intervention and Skills

Critical Reflection and Analysis

Knowledge

Rights, Justice and Economic Wellbeing

Diversity

Values and Ethics

Professionalism

Strategic Level

Advanced Level

Experienced Social Worker

Social Worker

ASYE

End Of Last Placement

End Of First Placement

Readiness For Direct Practice

Entry

HCPC Standards of Conduct, Performance & Ethics; Proficiency and CPD

SOCIAL WORK QUALIFYING PROGRAMMES

APPENDIX 2
THE CODE OF ETHICS FOR SOCIAL WORK – BRITISH ASSOCIATION OF SOCIAL WORKERS

Introduction – Scope and Objectives

The British Association of Social Workers is the professional association for social workers in the United Kingdom (UK). The Code of Ethics states the values and ethical principles on which the profession is based. The Association has a duty to ensure as far as possible that its members discharge their ethical obligations and are afforded the professional rights necessary for the safeguarding and promotion of the rights of people who use social work services. People who use social work services may be individuals (children, young people or adults), families or other groups or communities.

The Code is binding on all social workers who are BASW members in all roles, sectors and settings in the UK. Social workers have a responsibility to promote and work to the Code of Ethics in carrying out their obligations to people who use social work services, to their employers, to one another, to colleagues in other disciplines and to society. The Association commends and promotes the Code of Ethics to all social workers, educators and employers of social workers in the UK.

BASW's Code of Ethics, first adopted in 1975, has been revised and updated on several occasions. This Code of Ethics replaces the 2002 version. It takes as its starting point the internationally agreed *Definition of Social Work* (International Federation of Social Workers (IFSW) and International Association of Schools of Social Work (IASSW) (2000) and has also incorporated the international statement, *Ethics in Social Work – Statement of Principles* (IFSW and IASSW, 2004) with some revisions. These key documents were reviewed and agreed in 2010 by IFSW and IASSW.

Sections 1 and 2 of this document draw on the background, definition and statement of ethical principles of the IFSW/IASSW (2004) document, with amendments including the addition of 'professional integrity' as a value alongside human rights and social justice. Sections 3 comprises practice principles which indicate how the general ethical principles outlined in Section 2 should be put into practice in a UK context.

1. Background

1.1 Ethics in social work

Ethical awareness is fundamental to the professional practice of social workers. Their ability and commitment to act ethically is an essential aspect of the quality of the service offered to those who engage with social workers. Respect for human rights and a commitment to promoting social justice are at the core of social work practice throughout the world.

Social work grew out of humanitarian and democratic ideals, and its values are based on respect for the equality, worth, and dignity of all people. Since its beginnings over a century ago, social work practice has focused on meeting human needs and developing human potential. Human rights and social justice serve as the motivation and justification for social work action. In solidarity with those who are disadvantaged, the profession strives to alleviate poverty and to work with vulnerable and oppressed people in order to promote social inclusion. Social work values are embodied in the profession's national and international codes of ethics. Working definitions of ethics and values are given in the Appendix.

The Code comprises statements of values and ethical principles relating to human rights, social justice and professional integrity, followed by practice principles that indicate how the ethical principles should be applied in practice.

The practice principles are not intended to be exhaustive as some ethical challenges and problems facing social workers in practice are common and others are specific to particular countries and settings. The Code is not designed to provide a detailed set of rules about how social workers should act in specific situations or practice guidance. Rather, by outlining the general ethical principles, the aim is to encourage social workers across the UK to reflect on the challenges and dilemmas that face them and make ethically informed decisions about how to act in each particular case in accordance with the values of the profession.

Definition

Ethical problems often arise because social workers, for example:

- Work with conflicting interests and competing rights
- Have a role to support, protect and empower people, as well as having statutory duties and other obligations that may be coercive and restrict people's freedoms
- Are constrained by the availability of resources and institutional policies in society.

1.2 The international definition of social work

The social work profession promotes social change, problem solving in human relationships and the empowerment and liberation of people to enhance well-being. Utilising theories of human behaviour and social systems, social work intervenes at the points where people interact with their environments. Principles of human rights and social justice are fundamental to social work.

Social work in its various forms addresses the multiple, complex transactions between people and their environments. Its mission is to enable all people to develop their full potential, enrich their lives, and prevent dysfunction. Professional social work is focused on problem solving and change. As such, social workers are change agents in society and in the lives of the individuals, families and communities they serve. Social work is an interrelated system of values, theory and practice.

Theory:

Social work bases its methodology on a systematic body of evidence informed knowledge derived from research and practice evaluation, including local and indigenous knowledge specific to its context. It recognises the complexity of interactions between human beings and their environment, and the capacity of people both to be affected by and to alter the multiple influences upon them including biopsychosocial factors. The social work profession draws on theories of human development and behaviour and social systems to analyse complex situations and to facilitate individual, organisational, social and cultural changes.

Practice:

Social work practice addresses the barriers, inequities and injustices that exist in society. It responds to crises and emergencies as well as to everyday personal and social problems. Social work utilises a variety of skills, techniques, and activities consistent with its holistic focus on persons and their environments. Social work interventions range from primarily person-focused psychosocial processes to involvement in social policy, planning and development. These include counselling, clinical social work, group work, social pedagogical work, and family treatment and therapy as well as efforts to help people obtain services and resources in the community. Interventions also include agency administration, community organisation and engaging in social and political action to impact social policy and economic development. The holistic focus of social work is universal, but the priorities of social work practice will vary from country to country and from time to time depending on cultural, historical, legal and socio-economic conditions.

It is understood that social work in the 21st century is dynamic and evolving, and therefore no definition should be regarded as exhaustive.

2. Values and ethical principles

2.1 Human rights

Value

Social work is based on respect for the inherent worth and dignity of all people as expressed in the United Nations Universal Declaration of Human Rights (1948) and other related UN declarations on rights and the conventions derived from those declarations.

Principles

1 Upholding and promoting human dignity and well-being
Social workers should respect, uphold and defend each person's physical, psychological, emotional and spiritual integrity and well-being. They should work towards promoting the best interests of individuals and groups in society and the avoidance of harm.

2 Respecting the right to self-determination
Social workers should respect, promote and support people's dignity and right to make their own choices and decisions, irrespective of their values and life choices, provided this does not threaten the rights, safety and legitimate interests of others.

3 Promoting the right to participation
Social workers should promote the full involvement and participation of people using their services in ways that enable them to be empowered in all aspects of decisions and actions affecting their lives.

4 Treating each person as a whole

Social workers should be concerned with the whole person, within the family, community, societal and natural environments, and should seek to recognise all aspects of a person's life.

5 Identifying and developing strengths

Social workers should focus on the strengths of all individuals, groups and communities and thus promote their empowerment.

2.2 Social justice

Value

Social workers have a responsibility to promote social justice, in relation to society generally, and in relation to the people with whom they work.

Principles

1 Challenging discrimination

Social workers have a responsibility to challenge discrimination on the basis of characteristics such as ability, age, culture, gender or sex, marital status, socio-economic status, political opinions, skin colour, racial or other physical characteristics, sexual orientation or spiritual beliefs.

2 Recognising diversity

Social workers should recognise and respect the diversity of the societies in which they practise, taking into account individual, family, group and community differences.

3 Distributing resources

Social workers should ensure that resources at their disposal are distributed fairly, according to need.

4 Challenging unjust policies and practices

Social workers have a duty to bring to the attention of their employers, policy makers, politicians and the general public situations where resources are inadequate or where distribution of resources, policies and practice are oppressive, unfair, harmful or illegal.

5 Working in solidarity

Social workers, individually, collectively and with others have a duty to challenge social conditions that contribute to social exclusion, stigmatisation or subjugation, and work towards an inclusive society.

2.3 Professional integrity

Value

Social workers have a responsibility to respect and uphold the values and principles of the profession and act in a reliable, honest and trustworthy manner.

Principles

1 Upholding the values and reputation of the profession

Social workers should act at all times in accordance with the values and principles of the profession and ensure that their behaviour does not bring the profession into disrepute.

2 Being trustworthy

Social workers should work in a way that is honest, reliable and open, clearly explaining their roles, interventions and decisions and not seeking to deceive or manipulate people who use their services, their colleagues or employers.

3 Maintaining professional boundaries

Social workers should establish appropriate boundaries in their relationships with service users and colleagues, and not abuse their position for personal benefit, financial gain or sexual exploitation.

4 Making considered professional judgements

Social workers should make judgements based on balanced and considered reasoning, maintaining awareness of the impact of their own values, prejudices and conflicts of interest on their practice and on other people.

5 Being professionally accountable

Social workers should be prepared to account for and justify their judgements and actions to people who use services, to employers and the general public.

3. Ethical practice principles

Social workers have a responsibility to apply the professional values and principles set out above to their practice. They should act with integrity and treat people with compassion, empathy and care.

The ethical practice principles apply across the UK but they are not intended to be exhaustive or to constitute detailed prescription There will be variations in interpretation and guidance in the different countries. Social workers should take into account appropriate codes of practice, legislation, governance frameworks, professional practice and training standards in each UK country, provided they are consistent with the Code of Ethics. The Code is also supported by other BASW policy documents.

Social workers should strive to carry out the stated aims of their employers or commissioners, provided they are consistent with the Code of Ethics. BASW expects employers to have in place systems and approaches to promote a climate which supports, monitors, reviews and takes the necessary action to ensure social workers can comply with the Code of Ethics and other requirements to deliver safe and effective practice.

Principles

1 Developing professional relationships

Social workers should build and sustain professional relationships based on people's right to control their own lives and make their own choices and decisions. Social work relationships should be based on people's rights to respect, privacy, reliability and confidentiality. Social workers should communicate effectively and work in partnership with individuals, families, groups, communities and other agencies. They should value and respect the contribution of colleagues from other disciplines.

2 Assessing and managing risk

Social workers should recognise that people using social work services have the right to take risks and should enable them to identify and manage potential and actual risk, while seeking to ensure that their behaviour does not harm themselves or other people. Social workers should support people to reach informed decisions about their lives and promote their autonomy and independence, provided this does not conflict with their safety or with the rights of others. Social workers should only take actions which diminish people's civil or legal rights if it is ethically, professionally and legally justifiable.

3 Acting with the informed consent of service users, unless required by law to protect that person or another from risk of serious harm

Social workers should ascertain and respect, as far as possible, each individual's preferences, wishes and involvement in decision making, whether or not they or other persons have powers to make decisions on the person's behalf. This includes the duty to ascertain and respect a child's wishes and feelings, giving due weight to the child's maturity and understanding, where the law invests power of consent in respect of a child in the parent or guardian. Social workers need to acknowledge the impact of their own informal and coercive power and that of the organisations involved.

4 Providing information

Social workers should give people the information they need to make informed choices and decisions. They should enable people to access all information recorded about themselves, subject to any limitations imposed by law. Social workers should assist people to understand and exercise their rights including making complaints and other remedies.

5 Sharing information appropriately

Social workers should ensure the sharing of information is subject to ethical requirements in respect of privacy and confidentiality across agencies and professions, and within a multi-purpose agency.

6 Using authority in accordance with human rights principles

Social workers should use the authority of their role in a responsible, accountable and respectful manner. They should exercise authority appropriately to safeguard people with whom they work and to ensure people have as much control over their lives as is consistent with the rights of others.

7 Empowering people

Social workers should promote and contribute to the development of positive policies, procedures and practices which are anti-oppressive and empowering. They should respect people's beliefs, values, culture, goals, needs, preferences, relationships and affiliations. Social workers should recognise their own prejudices to ensure they do not discriminate against any person or group. They should ensure that services are offered and delivered in a culturally appropriate manner. They should challenge and seek to address any actions of colleagues who demonstrate negative discrimination or prejudice.

8 Challenging the abuse of human rights

Social workers should be prepared to challenge discriminatory, ineffective and unjust policies, procedures and practice. They should challenge the abuse of power and the exclusion of people from decisions that affect them. Social workers should not collude with the erosion of human rights or allow their skills to be used for inhumane purposes such as systematic abuse, detention of child asylum seekers and threats to family life of those in vulnerable positions.

9 Being prepared to whistleblow

Social workers should be prepared to report bad practice using all available channels including complaints procedures and if necessary use public interest disclosure legislation and whistleblowing guidelines.

10 Maintaining confidentiality

Social workers should respect the principles of confidentiality that apply to their relationships and ensure that confidential information is only divulged with the consent of the person using social work services or the informant. Exceptions to this may only be justified on the basis of a greater ethical requirement such as evidence of serious risk or the preservation of life. Social workers need to explain the nature of that confidentiality to people with whom they work and any circumstances where confidentiality must be waived should be made explicit. Social workers should identify dilemmas about confidentiality and seek support to address these issues.

11 Maintaining clear and accurate records

Social workers should maintain clear, impartial and accurate records and provision of evidence to support professional judgements. They should record only relevant matters and specify the source of information.

12 Striving for objectivity and self-awareness in professional practice

Social workers should reflect and critically evaluate their practice and be aware of their impact on others. Social workers should recognise the limits of their practice and seek advice or refer to another professional if necessary to ensure they work in a safe and effective manner.

13 Using professional supervision and peer support to reflect on and improve practice

Social workers should take responsibility for ensuring they have access to professional supervision and discussion which supports them to reflect and make sound professional judgements based on good practice. BASW expects all employers to provide appropriate professional supervision for social workers and promote effective team work and communication.

14 Taking responsibility for their own practice and continuing professional development

Social workers should develop and maintain the attitudes, knowledge, understanding and skills to provide quality services and accountable practice. They need to keep up to date with relevant research, learning from other professionals and service users. BASW expects employers to ensure social workers' learning and development needs are met and seek adequate resources to do so.

15 Contributing to the continuous improvement of professional practice

Social workers should strive to create conditions in employing agencies and in their countries where the principles of the Code are discussed, evaluated and upheld in practice. They should engage in ethical debate with their colleagues and employers to share knowledge and take responsibility for making ethically informed decisions. They should endeavour to seek changes in policies, procedures, improvements to services or working conditions as guided by the ethics of the profession.

16 Taking responsibility for the professional development of others

Social workers should contribute to the education and training of colleagues and students by sharing knowledge and practice wisdom. They should identify, develop, use and disseminate knowledge, theory and practice. They should contribute to social work education, including the provision of good quality placements, and ensure students are informed of their ethical responsibilities to use the Code in their practice.

17 Facilitating and contributing to evaluation and research

Social workers should use professional knowledge and experience to engage in research and to contribute to the development of ethically based policy and programmes. They should analyse and evaluate the quality and outcomes of their practice with people who use social work services.

Appendix Some working definitions of key terms

(adapted from Banks, S. (2012) *Ethics and Values in Social Work*, 4th edition, Basingstoke, Palgrave Macmillan, BASW Macmillan Practical Social Work Series)

Working definitions of ethics and professional ethics

Broadly speaking, 'ethics' is about matters of right and wrong conduct, good and bad qualities of character and responsibilities attached to relationships. Although the subject matter of ethics is often said to be human welfare, the bigger picture also includes the flourishing of animals and the whole ecosystem. The term 'ethics' may be used in a singular sense to refer to the study of right and wrong norms of behaviour, good and bad qualities of character; or in a plural sense, to refer to the actual norms and qualities.

Professional ethics concerns matters of right and wrong conduct, good and bad qualities of character and the professional responsibilities attached to relationships in a work context.

Working definitions of values and social work values

In everyday usage, 'values' is often used to refer to one or all of religious, moral, cultural, political or ideological beliefs, principles, attitudes, opinions or preferences. In social work, 'values' can be regarded as particular types of beliefs that people hold about what is regarded as worthy or valuable. In the context of professional practice, the use of the term 'belief' reflects the status that values have as stronger than mere opinions or preferences.

The term 'social work values' refers to a range of beliefs about what is regarded as worthy or valuable in a social work context (general beliefs about the nature of the good society, general principles about how to achieve this through actions, and the desirable qualities or character traits of professional practitioners).

Principles and standards (or rules)

Principles are essential norms in a system of thought or belief, which form the basis of reasoning in that system. In codes of ethics principles are often divided into two kinds:

Ethical principles – general statements of ethical principles underpinning the work, relating to attitudes, rights and duties about human welfare, for example: 'respect for the autonomy of service users'; 'promotion of human welfare'.

Principles of professional practice – general statements about how to achieve what is intended for the good of the service user, for example: 'collaboration with colleagues'.

Principles have a much broader scope than rules (or 'standards'), tending to apply to all people in all circumstances (although in the case of social work, principles often refer to 'all service users'). So, for example, 'social workers should respect the autonomy of service users' is an ethical principle; whereas, 'social workers should not disclose confidential information to third-party payers unless clients have authorised such disclosure' might be regarded as an ethical standard or rule. Standards can also be divided into two kinds, although often they are not clearly distinguished in codes of ethics:

Ethical standards or rules – some general 'do's and don'ts', sometimes framed as 'standards' for example: 'do not permit knowledge to be used for discriminatory policies'; 'protect all confidential information'.

Professional practice standards – very specific guidance relating to professional practice, for example: 'declare a bequest in a client's will'; 'advertising should not claim superiority'.

PDF copies of this document are downloadable at:
www.basw.co.uk

Copyright © British Association of Social Workers
All rights reserved.

No part of this publication may be reproduced in any material form without the written permission of the copyright owner.

INDEX

*9 7 8 1 4 0 8 2 5 2 5 3 6 *

An environmentally friendly book printed and bound in England by www.printondemand-worldwide.com

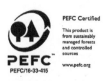

PEFC Certified

This product is
from sustainably
managed forests
and controlled
sources

PEFC™

www.pefc.org

PEFC/16-33-415

This book is made of chain-of-custody materials; FSC materials for the cover and PEFC materials for the text pages.

#0411 - 101115 - C162 - 240/170/9 - PB - 9781408252536